GUT HEALTH HACKS THAT WORK

SAFE GUT HEALTH HACKS FOR WOMEN

VANESSA ALVAREZ

CONTENTS

CHAPTER 1
WHY YOUR GUT HEALTH MIGHT BE KILLING YOU

YOUR GUT HEALTH is important because it affects every aspect of your life. Your gut health directly impacts your brain function, mood, energy level, immune system, weight management, digestion, skin health, and overall well-being. If your gut isn't healthy, you're not getting enough vitamins and minerals, which means you're not getting the energy you need to live a happy life. And when your gut isn't healthy...your brain doesn't work right, your skin looks terrible, your moods fluctuate, and your immune system is weak.

Unfortunately, many women suffer from poor gut health. This includes bloating, constipation, diarrhea, gas, and other gastrointestinal problems. Poor gut health can be caused by stress, diet, antibiotics, and other factors.

Let's Talk About Women's Gut Health: The Importance of Hormones, Digestion and More

Did you know that your gut is connected to your brain? While most people tend to think of the brain as being in charge of the body, the gut plays a large role in almost everything we do. The second largest organ in the human body, the gut is home to trillions of bacteria. These bacteria are known as the microbiome, and the vast majority of them reside in the small intestine. When we talk about gut health, we're usually referring to the health of the digestive system—the large intestine and the colon. The health of the gut plays an important role in our general wellbeing. If the gut is healthy, we will have high levels of good bacteria. But if the gut is unhealthy, the other way around. The good bacteria in the gut will outnumber the bad bacteria, and this will have a positive effect on our overall health. In this article, we'll be exploring the gut, its importance, and how the health of the female gut can be improved.

Factors That Can Affect Gut Health in Women

The gut is influenced by a wide range of environmental and genetic factors that can affect its health. These factors can be divided into two categories: the "abdominal" and the "external." The "external" factors include diet, stress, and other lifestyle habits, while the "internal" factors include our genetics, age, and medical history.

Gut Health and Women's Health

The gut plays an important role in women's health. A healthy gut can affect a woman's ability to maintain a healthy weight, prevent disease, and improve overall wellbeing. The gut has a direct connection to the brain, which is why the health of your gut can have a significant impact on your brain function.

The Female Gut is Different from the Male Gut

The gut microbiota is influenced by hormones that are unique to women. This includes hormones that regulate metabolism, the immune system, and digestive function. The female gut contains different bacterial species than the male gut. Some of these bacteria are related to metabolism and weight management, while others are related to reproduction, the immune system, and digestion. Many women have a healthy gut microbiota, but still struggle with weight issues and/or chronic digestive issues.

Sex hormones have a large impact on the gut microbiome of women. This includes hormones that regulate metabolism, the immune system, and digestive function. The female gut contains different bacterial species than the male gut. Some of these bacteria are related to metabolism and weight management, while others are related to reproduction, the immune system, and digestion. Many women have a healthy gut microbiota, but still struggle with weight issues and/or chronic digestive issues.

The Importance of Good Bacteria for Women's Health

The gut microbiota can have a significant impact on women's health. There are many ways in which our gut microbiota plays an important role in our health.

- Good bacteria can prevent the development of certain diseases. A healthy gut microbiota can prevent the development of certain diseases, such as inflammatory bowel disease and metabolic diseases.
- It can affect our ability to maintain a healthy weight. This is often referred to as "weight loss resistance," and is the main focus of the novel "metagenomics" technology.
- It can affect our mood and our ability to stay focused. This has to do with the "gut-brain axis" —the gut's connection to the brain. The good bacteria in the gut can have a significant impact on the health of the female brain, which is especially relevant during pregnancy.
- It can affect our metabolism. The gut microbiota, and in particular the bacteria in the "enterotype" of your gut, can have a significant impact on your metabolism.

Folate and Women's Health

Folate is a B vitamin found in many plant-based foods, such as green leafy vegetables, legumes, and fruit. Folate is required for the production of proteins, and is especially important in women as it is critical to fetal development. Deficiency in folate can lead to poor health in several ways. It can affect your ability to reproduce, it can lead to birth defects, or it can negatively affect your metabolism.

Proteins in Gut Health

Proteins are made up of chains of amino acids, which are building blocks for the formation of enzymes, hormones, and antibodies. Proteins play a key role in gut health.

Your ability to digest and absorb proteins depends on the size, shape, and structure of the protein. If you're not able to break down the protein properly, you won't be able to absorb it. Proteins are found in a variety of foods, but they are most abundant in protein-containing foods like eggs, dairy, meat, fish, and nuts. It's important to keep in mind that protein digestion is dependent on the health of your gut.

Hormones and the Female Gut

The hormones produced by the gut microbiota are known as "enteric hormones." These hormones have been shown to have a huge impact on a woman's health, and can be divided into two categories: metabolic and immunomodulatory.

The metabolic hormones produced by the microbiota play a key role in maintaining a healthy weight, by regulating the levels of various gut metabolites. The immunomodulatory hormones produced by the gut microbiota have been shown to have a protective effect on the body.

Digestion and the Female Gut

Let's first talk a little bit about digestion and the gut. When you eat a meal, food particles are broken down by digestive enzymes into small fragments. These fragments then enter the small intestine and are absorbed by the cells in the wall of the intestine. The substances absorbed from the intestine then enter the blood stream and are delivered to the rest of the body. The small intestine contains several types of cells. Some of these cells have a very selective ability to absorb only certain substances, such as sugars and amino acids. The substances that are not absorbed by the small intestine are removed in the large intestine, either through the stool or through the colon, where bacteria break down the substances into their constituent parts.

The female gut has special mechanisms for the digestion of specific nutrients. There are two main types of pathways in the gut, and they are both responsible for breaking down proteins: the "pathway of digestion" and the "pathway of absorption." The "pathway of digestion" is the pathway that breaks down proteins in the small intestine. The small intestine is lined with microvillus structures, which are also known as "proβ-defensins."

These defensins are responsible for the breakdown of proteins in the small intestine, and they do this by producing hydrogen peroxide.

The Role of Stress in Gut Health

Stress can affect the health of the gut in a variety of ways. For example, chronic stress can lead to changes in gut hormones, causing the gut microbiota to become unbalanced, and this can lead to inflammation within the gut. Chronic stress can also disrupt gut-brain signalling and cause changes in the gut through both the central nervous system and the enteric nervous system. Chronic stress has been shown to alter the bacteria in the gut, leading to an overgrowth of enteric pathogens that can invade the blood stream and cause systemic infections.

The Hormones Play a Role in Gut Health

When it comes to hormones, the gut and the brain are connected. Among other things, the gut and the brain communicate through hormones. The gut contains a number of hormone-producing cells, called enteric nervous system neurons, that connect directly to the central nervous system. These neurons contain a number of important neurotransmitters and neurohormones that have a direct impact on the gut. These include serotonin, dopamine and opioids—all of which play a part in gut function.

What's the Difference Between Gut Health and Bowel Health?

Gut health is the overall wellbeing of the gut and its cells. It includes good bacteria, the function of the nervous system and the function of the intestinal cells. Bacterial balance is a much narrower term that refers to the number of good bacteria present in the gut. While bacteria can be added to the gut, it's actually impossible to take away bacteria from the gut. The gut has been compared to a 'microbiome-rich battleground', but the bacteria in the gut are actually a more important part of human health than previously thought. The bacteria in the gut are known as the gut microbiome. The microbiome plays an essential role in human health, including the production of vitamins, the development of the immune system, and the metabolism of food.

Microbiomes and the female gut

The digestive system of a woman is very different from that of a man. The majority of bacteria in a man's gut is known as 'flora masculine'. In a woman, on the other hand, the majority of bacteria is 'flora feminine'. The gut microbiome is one of the most important aspects of female gut health and can be greatly influenced by diet and lifestyle. The balance and diversity of gut flora is important for several reasons. Consider this: the human body is largely made up of 10–20% bacteria, and if the bacteria are out of balance, then the human body is also affected. Important aspects of female gut health that can be affected by gut flora include the following:

The female gut is an ecosystem of microbes like nowhere else in the human body. The health of the gut is a reflection of the health of the body, and it can be greatly affected by diet, lifestyle, and even mental health. The female gut microbiota is uniquely adapted to women's metabolic needs and is also responsive to the hormones that regulate the reproductive system. Gut health is important for a variety of reasons. The health of the gut can be affected by stress, diet, and lifestyle, and can also be used as an indicator of mental health and wellbeing. The female gut microbiota is uniquely adapted to women's metabolic needs, and is also responsive to the hormones that regulate the reproductive system.

Symptoms Of An Unhealthy Gut That You Might Be Ignoring

Do you ever feel tired all the time? Or do you ever feel depressed? Or do you ever feel anxious? Or do you ever have trouble processing your emotions? If you answered yes to one or more of these questions, you might be suffering from an unhealthy gut. A healthy gut plays an important role in keeping your body functioning optimally. When your gut is healthy, it can handle food and other substances you ingest. When your gut is unhealthy, it can lead to a variety of symptoms. In this blog post, we'll explore some of the most common signs that your gut is unhealthy and how you can get back on track.

Irritable Bowel Syndrome

Irritable bowel syndrome, or IBS, is a condition characterized by chronic abdominal pain that can occur in several forms, including cramping pain, bloating, and gas. The cause of IBS is unknown, but one possible trigger is an unhealthy gut. If you're experiencing abdominal discomfort, it's important to get evaluated by your doctor. You can also try some simple gut-healing strategies to get your gut back in shape. First, make sure you're drinking enough water. Water is essential for digestion, and not drinking enough can lead to constipation and other gut issues. Eating fiber-rich foods, such as whole grains, beans, and fruits, can also help you get moving efficiently.

Depression

Stress can wreak havoc on your gut and lead to an unhealthy gut. In fact, it's been shown in several studies that gut issues are correlated with anxiety and depression. A healthy gut is essential for mental health. Your gut plays an important role in processing nutrition, vitamins, and minerals you consume through your diet. When your gut is unhealthy, it can lead to a variety of symptoms, including poor mental health. When your gut is healthy, you can better process the nutrients that make up your diet, including vitamins and minerals. An unhealthy gut can interfere with this process, leading to symptoms of poor mental health, such as depression.

Sleep Problems

When your gut is unhealthy, you may wake up in the middle of the night with gas and bloating or abdominal pain. If you're struggling to fall asleep, you might try taking a relaxing bath or drinking herbal tea before bed. Sleep disturbances are one of the most common symptoms of an unhealthy gut. Lack of sleep can lead to moodiness, low energy, and an inability to focus. If you're having trouble sleeping, it's important to work with your doctor to rule out any medical causes. Additionally, a healthy gut can improve sleep quality by creating the ideal environment for rest. According to one study, people with gut issues often had a lack of certain amino acids in their diets, which affected their sleep. You can get these amino acids by eating a protein-rich diet and taking a high-quality amino acid supplement, such as Source Naturals Proprietary Blend.

Anxiety and Panic Attacks

A healthy gut is essential for processing anxiety and other mental illnesses. According to one study, people who have anxiety often have an unhealthy gut, with low gut levels of certain nutrients, including zinc and B vitamins. What can you do if you have anxiety or panic attacks? First, it's important to rule out any medical causes. You can discuss this with your doctor, who can conduct a thorough physical exam and blood test to rule out any underlying causes. If your gut is healthy and you don't have a medical cause for your anxiety, it may be because you're consuming foods that contribute to anxiety. Eating a diet high in sugar and white flour, and low in fruits, vegetables, and other foods that are high in vitamins and minerals, can lead to feelings of anxiety. To address this, you can try forming a food plan and trying some of the strategies we discuss in our blog post on What To Eat When You Have Anxiety.

Autoimmune Disorders

Autoimmune disorders are conditions in which your immune system attacks your own body, including your gut. The most common autoimmune disorders are inflammatory bowel disease, Celiac disease, and Hashimoto's thyroiditis. A healthy gut is essential for preventing autoimmune disorders. Feeding your gut the right foods can prevent it from being inflamed, which can lead to various auto-immune disorders. In order to feed your gut the right foods, we all need to adjust our eating behaviors. For example, we should all be eating more vegetables and fruits, which are high in vitamins and minerals, and low in sugar. We should also be eating smaller portions of protein and carbs.

You're Constipated

Constipation is a common symptom of an unhealthy gut. According to one study, people with constipation often have an unhealthy gut. What can you do if you're suffering from constipation? First, you should make sure you're drinking enough water. As we discussed above, water is essential for digestion. Second, you can try eating more fiber-rich foods, such as whole grains, beans, and fruits. You can also try some simple gut-healing strategies, such as taking a probiotic supplement, practicing yoga, or doing gentle movement, such as walking or walking meditation.

You Have Acid Reflux

Acid reflux occurs when stomach acid flows back up into your esophagus, causing heartburn and other symptoms. If you're experiencing heartburn regularly or if you're wondering if you might have acid reflux, it's important to get evaluated by your doctor. Acid reflux is often a sign of an unhealthy gut. What can you do if you have acid reflux? First, you should make sure you're drinking enough water. As we discussed above, water is essential for digestion. Second, you can try eating more fiber-rich foods, such as whole grains, beans, and fruits. You can also try some simple gut-healing strategies, such as taking probiotics or eating ginger.

You Have Food Sensitivities

Food sensitivities are a common sign of an unhealthy gut. According to one study, people with allergies often have an unhealthy gut. What can you do if you suspect you have a food sensitivity? First, you should make sure you're drinking enough water. As we discussed above, water is essential for digestion. Second, you can try eating more fiber-rich foods, such as whole grains, beans, and fruits. You can also try some simple gut-healing strategies, such as taking probiotics or eating ginger. You can also try elimination diets, which help identify problematic foods. For example, if you suspect you're sensitive to gluten, you can try eliminating gluten from your diet for a few weeks and see how you feel.

Leaky Gut

In modern Western society, it's common to suffer from a condition called "leaky gut." According to one doctor, "Gut leakiness is a common consequence of a poor diet and is the result of undigested food particles making their way into the bloodstream through a breach in the gut barrier. When this happens, the immune system becomes activated and tries to rid the body of these foreign particles, often through inflammation." A healthy gut plays an important role in keeping your body functioning optimally. When your gut is unhealthy, it can lead to a variety of symptoms, including poor mental health. We all need a healthy gut to live a happy, productive life.

Overweight

From a diet perspective, a diet high in sugar and fat is not good for your gut. According to one study, people with a "Western-style diet" (a diet high in sugar, refined grains, and processed foods) often have an unhealthy gut. What can you do if you have an unhealthy gut that's leading to weight gain? First, you should make sure you're drinking enough water. As we discussed above, water is essential for digestion. Second, you can try eating more fiber-rich foods, such as whole grains, beans, and fruits.

According to the CDC, more than one-third of Americans are obese, and that number is expected to rise. Obesity is a gut issue. Over time, your gut might have developed a hypersensitivity to certain nutrients, leading to an unhealthy gut. This hypersensitivity might make you feel hungry when you're not supposed to be, or it might make you feel full even when you don't need to be. If you're overweight and you're not sure why, your gut health might be part of the reason. In order to lose weight, you might need to treat your gut health first.

Brain Fog

Brain fog is a common sign of poor gut health. Brain fog occurs when the brain doesn't get enough nutrients, which can lead to a variety of symptoms. Poor gut health can affect your brain function in several ways. If your gut isn't healthy, you might be feeling: anxiety, brain fog, constitutional symptoms, constant fatigue, constant hunger, constant brain fog, constant bloating, constant nausea, constant low mood, Crohn's, depression, difficulty concentrating, eczema, fatigue, fibromyalgia, headaches, indigestion, insomnia, low libido, muddled thinking, muscle tension, nervous system issues, poor digestion, psoriasis, psoriatic arthritis, poor memory, psoriasis, psoriatic arthritus, psoriatic arthritis, puffy eyes, recurring infections, restlessness, stress, uncontrollable urges, undereating, and more.

Other Signs of an Unhealthy Gut

Other signs of an unhealthy gut include: chronic infections, depression, eczema, low libido, psoriasis, psoriatic arthritis, and more. The good news is that most of these signs can be reversed with a healthy gut. If you're suffering from any of these signs, it's important to get your gut health back on track. To do this, you can start by eliminating processed foods, eating more fibrous vegetables, drinking lots of water, and taking a fiber supplement. These three things can help get your gut health on track in no time.

CHAPTER 2
HOW TO RECOVER YOUR GUT HEALTH

Everyone knows that maintaining a balanced, healthy diet is essential to staying happy and healthy. But what if your gut is sending you mixed signals, and you're not sure how to respond? Many of us are familiar with the term 'gut health' - we know it's important, but we may not know exactly why. Your gut, also known as your 'second brain' or 'gastrointestinal tract,' can seem like a complicated place — but it's worth exploring to discover what benefits there are to having a strong and healthy gut. Read on for 10 ways that you can boost your gut health.

Eat prebiotic foods

Prebiotic foods, such as asparagus, artichokes, or bananas, are known for being 'fermentable' — an important concept to understand in terms of gut health. Fermentation happens naturally in the gut, and is a process that breaks down food and turns it into beneficial nutrients. There's a diverse range of probiotic foods, most of which are also rich in fiber — another key part of a healthy gut. While many people are aware that bananas are high in fiber, they may not realize that they're also prebiotic — meaning that they're likely to help support your gut health. Other prebiotic-rich foods include legumes, garlic, oats, and asparagus.

Add more fiber to your diet

Fiber is an essential part of any healthy diet, but many of us don't get enough. It's important to note, however, that we don't need to get all our fiber from our food. Supplements such as psyllium husks or soluble fiber can also help to improve your gut health. When it comes to fiber, the more you eat, the better — but don't go overboard; too much fiber can cause bloating and other digestive issues. The recommended daily intake of fiber is around 20-30 grams for women and 30-40 grams for men — but the best way to find out what's right for you is to speak to a nutritionist. If you're new to adding fiber to your diet, start off slowly. A good rule of thumb is to gradually increase your fiber intake by 5 grams each week until you reach your goal.

Exercise regularly

Regular exercise is another key part of a healthy diet, and it's just as important for your gut health as it is for your heart and muscles. When you exercise regularly, it stimulates your digestive system, helping to move your food through your gut — and, as a result, preventing constipation. Exercise also helps to relieve stress, which can be another factor in digestive issues. When you exercise, your body releases endorphins, which are hormones that naturally reduce stress and help you to feel calmer and more relaxed. When you feel less stressed, it's much easier to avoid digestive issues, such as irritable bowel syndrome (IBS).

Consume probiotic foods and supplements

Fermented foods like yoghurt, kefir, kimchi, or sauerkraut are rich in probiotics — microorganisms that are essential for a healthy gut. Probiotics can be a great addition to your diet, or you can also take a supplement. Some experts recommend that all adults take a probiotic supplement once a day — and it's particularly important for people who are at risk of digestive issues, including pregnant women and those who experience travel sickness. When you choose the best probiotic supplements for you, be sure to read the label. Ideally, you want to find a product that has around 10-20 billion colony-forming units (CFUs). It's also important to note that there are two types of probiotics — living, and 'dead' or 'heat-killed.'

Get enough vitamin D

Vitamin D is known as the 'sunshine vitamin' because we can also get it from a healthy diet — and it's important for your gut health. A Vitamin D deficiency is associated with an increased risk of IBD, as well as other digestive issues. A Vitamin D deficiency may also affect the health of your gut. Certain types of probiotics, such as lactobacilli, rely on vitamin D to establish themselves in your gut. If you're not getting enough sunlight or you're not eating foods rich in vitamin D, such as fish or eggs, you should consider taking a daily supplement. Other nutrients that are also important for gut health include iron, zinc, and magnesium.

Try relaxation techniques

When you're stressed, your digestive system is more likely to become upset — which can lead to uncomfortable symptoms such as bloating, constipation, or diarrhea. Stress can also slow down your digestive system, meaning that your food may not be fully digested and metabolized. There are many different ways in which you can reduce your stress levels, including meditation, yoga, or even going for a walk in nature. You may also find that getting enough sleep, practicing good time management, and reducing your caffeine intake can help to alleviate your stress levels — and, in turn, improve your gut health.

Watch what you eat — and what you drink

As well as eating a healthy diet, it's also important to avoid certain foods that may upset your gut. Food allergies, intolerances, and sensitivities can all cause issues for your digestive system, so look out for common culprits including gluten, dairy, and eggs. It's also important to be careful about the drinks that you consume. When you're feeling under the weather, it's tempting to reach for the caffeine-rich soft drink — but these drinks are high in sugar and can actually slow down your digestive system. Instead, opt for water, herbal teas, or warm milk.

CHAPTER 3
HOW TO TEST YOUR GUT HEALTH AT HOME

GUT HEALTH AFFECTS a lot more than just your digestion. A healthy gut means your body is able to digest food well, it keeps bad bacteria out of your system, and it creates helpful compounds that keep you from getting sick. In a perfect world, everyone would have excellent gut health. But in reality, most people are dealing with poor gut health—and it's not something you want to ignore. It's been linked to everything from asthma and allergies to autoimmune disorders and chronic diseases like diabetes and obesity. Luckily, there are plenty of ways you can test your gut health and see how you can improve it right now. These eight tips will help you get started on the path to a healthier digestive system today!

Eat prebiotic foods

Prebiotics are basically foods that help your gut bacteria grow and thrive. They're not the same as probiotic foods like yogurt that contain active cultures. But they're still really important for your gut health. Prebiotic foods include apples, artichokes, asparagus, bananas, beets, broccoli, Brussels sprouts, carrots, cantaloupe, Chinese cabbage, foods made with inulin, garlic, leeks, onions, olives, oregano, plantain, rhubarb, rye, sage, sea vegetables, taro, and yacon root. Prebiotics are especially important if you're taking a probiotic supplement. Taking probiotics can help your gut by bringing more good bacteria into your system. But it can also cause your system to expel the bad bacteria you don't want. If you aren't also eating prebiotic foods, then the good bacteria you take in won't be able to grow.

Take a probiotic supplement

Taking a probiotic supplement is a great way to restore balance to your gut. It'll help you add more good bacteria to your system, which will promote digestion and keep you from getting sick. The best probiotics for gut health come in capsules or powdered form. They're marked as "live cultures" and "germ-free" to make sure they're safe for your system. Prebiotics and probiotics can be taken together. It's best to talk to your doctor about what dosage is best for your health situation.

Test your stool

If you're curious about your gut health, you can actually test your stool to see what's going on inside your system. There are a few different stool tests that can give you insight into your gut health. Stool analysis is used to check for bacteria and parasites in your system. You can get it done at your doctor's office or at any lab that offers stool testing. If you're trying to find out if you have too much or too little fiber in your system, you can get a test called a fiber stool test. This will give you a breakdown of how much fiber you're eating.

Monitor your diet

If you're having digestive issues, you may want to keep a food journal to see if there's a pattern. Food journals are a great way to figure out what's going on with your system. You can use an app to track things like how much you're eating, how often you're eating, and what types of foods you're eating. You can also use a journal to track how your system is feeling. Are you more gassy than usual? Arc you feeling more bloated? Are you having trouble digesting certain foods? This information can help you narrow down what's going wrong in your gut and which foods could be causing issues.

Try an elimination diet

This might seem extreme, but if you're really struggling with poor gut health, an elimination diet might be worth trying. An elimination diet is exactly what it sounds like—you eliminate potential triggers for a certain period of time to see if that changes your system. While this isn't sound medical advice, it can be a good way to determine what foods are causing you issues. You can visit a dietitian if you want help designing a good elimination diet. Eliminating certain foods can also help you see what your gut health is like without those foods. It can help you identify problem areas in your system that you might not have noticed before.

Get fasted stool testing done

When you eat, your body uses a lot of your energy to digest and break down the food you're consuming. That can make it harder to examine your stool and see what's going on in your gut. Eating a meal before you take a sample of your stool will help you get a more accurate reading. You can try taking a sample right after you wake up in the morning. You'll have a full 12 hours to eliminate your food before you collect your sample at the end of the day. This is called a "fasted stool test" and it can be done at home. You can even do it in the bathroom—we promise we won't judge! A fasted stool test can help you identify bacteria and parasites in your system that a normal stool test might not pick up on.

Try infrared sauna therapy

Infrared sauna therapy has been shown to improve gut health by boosting circulation, improving immunity, and breaking down toxins that can cause digestive issues. This is especially helpful if you're dealing with IBS or you've recently taken antibiotics that can mess with your system. There are many different types of infrared saunas on the market. But research indicates that they're not all equal, so you want to make sure you're getting a high-quality product to get the results you want.

Ask your doctor for a fecal microbiota test (FMIT)

You might have heard of a "stool test" but what you might not know is that there are actually two different types of stool tests. You can get a "stool test" or a "fecal microbiota test." The latter is actually a better way to look at your gut health because it examines the bacteria in your stool and not just the amount of fiber or nutrients. Fecal microbiota testing (or FMIT for short) is the gold standard for gut health. You provide a sample of your stool and get tested for everything from bacteria to parasites. Your digestive system is an important part of your health. Taking care of it should be a priority for everyone. And these eight tips can help you learn ways to improve your gut health and keep your digestive system running smoothly.

CHAPTER 4

GUT HEALTH AND MENTAL HEALTH: THE LINK IS MORE THAN YOU KNOW!

MENTAL HEALTH and the gut are two issues that aren't often discussed together. While it may not be common knowledge, the link between gastrointestinal health and mental health is becoming more recognized by researchers, clinicians, and individuals. The gut is a major player when it comes to mental health. The gastrointestinal tract has its own nervous system called the "enteric nervous system." This system has as many neurons as the spinal cord in your back, but it's all located in your stomach and intestines! As scientists learn more about this connection, there are new ways that we can treat mental illness with a focus on improving digestive health. In this blog post, we explore the connection between gut health and mental health—and how you can have healthy guts to improve your mental well-being.

What Does Gut Health Have to Do With Mental Health?

Healthy digestion is essential to having a healthy brain. If you experience digestive issues, your body will have trouble absorbing the nutrients it needs to function properly. When your body lacks important nutrients, your brain function will suffer. Gut health problems such as irritable bowel syndrome, inflammatory bowel disease, and chronic constipation can lead to poor mental health. The gut bacteria can also affect mental health in various ways. For example, certain bacteria in your gut can produce neurotransmitters that affect your mood and emotions. Furthermore, when the gut is inflamed, it can negatively impact the brain through the nervous system of the gut. When your gut isn't working properly, you could experience symptoms such as gas, bloating, nausea, abdominal pain, and even more serious issues like blood in your stool. These can be signs that something is wrong in your gut, and if left untreated, can cause more serious long-term damage.

Depression and Anxiety and Their Link to the Gut

There is a connection between depression and the gut. The condition of your digestive system can have an impact on your mood and emotions. Poor gut health can leave you fatigued, irritable, and anxious. On the other hand, a healthy gut can make you feel more positive and happier. When the gut is inflamed or not functioning properly, the body produces more cortisol. Cortisol is the stress hormone that can leave you feeling anxious, tired, and depressed. This can lead to a vicious cycle—poor gut health can cause your mood to suffer, and vice versa.

Irritable Bowel Syndrome and Its Link to Mental Health

Another gastrointestinal disorder that can affect mental health is irritable bowel syndrome (IBS). Individuals with IBS have a higher risk of developing mood disorders such as anxiety and depression. However, there is no clear answer as to why IBS and mental health are linked. It may be due to the fact that individuals with IBS are often prescribed antidepressants to help manage their symptoms.

Constipation and Its Link to Mental Illness

Constipation can also lead to anxiety and depression. The more often you are constipated, the more toxins build up in your body, making you feel sluggish and depressed. When the bowels are not working properly, toxins are not being removed from the body. This can lead to the build-up of serious issues, such as intestinal permeability. Intestinal permeability, also known as "leaky gut", can lead to a wide range of health issues, including mental health issues such as anxiety and depression. Intestinal permeability occurs when the gut is inflamed, and the barrier between your digestive tract and your bloodstream is broken down. When this

happens, toxins and bacteria leak into your bloodstream, which can negatively impact your mental health
and other organs in the body.

When your gut is healthy and functioning properly, you
will be less likely to experience mental health symptoms
such as anxiety and depression. Eating a balanced diet
that includes fermented foods, probiotics, prebiotics,
and fiber can be beneficial for mental health. Furthermore, taking care of your gut by making sure you stay
hydrated, get enough sleep, and avoid stress will help
keep your digestive system operating at its best. This will
leave you feeling happier, healthier, and more
energized.

CHAPTER 5
ALL YOU NEED TO KNOW ABOUT FOOD INTOLERANCE AND GUT HEALTH

FOOD INTOLERANCE IS NOT a new topic in the world of nutrition. However, there has recently been a spike in its visibility and prevalence. The reason for this is that food intolerances are actually very common conditions. In fact, around one third of the world's population experiences some form of food intolerance at some point in their lives. However, many people are still not aware of it and this can be quite problematic. Uncontrolled or undiagnosed food intolerance can have negative effects on your general health, causing issues like bloating, stomach aches, fatigue, headaches, and much more. Luckily, by reading this article you will know everything you need to know about food intolerance and gut health so that you can take measures to prevent any further issues.

What is Food Intolerance?

Food intolerance is basically an adverse reaction to certain foods. These adverse reactions are not caused by allergy, but by a negative metabolic reaction. Food intolerances cause adverse reactions to certain foods and beverages such as coffee, alcohol, vinegar, and citrus fruits. The symptoms of food intolerance are not the same for everyone, and are often different for each individual. Some of the most common signs of food intolerance include bloating, stomach aches, diarrhea, gas, fatigue, headaches, and skin rashes. However, many people with food intolerance may not experience any of these symptoms, which is why it is important to be aware of other signs, too. You may have food intolerance if you notice that you have digestive issues such as bloating, gas, diarrhea, or constipation after eating a certain food. If a certain food makes you feel tired, moody, or have a headache, you might have food intolerance, too. Food intolerance can also affect your mental health and can cause anxiety, panic attacks, and depression. Food intolerance can also be a sign of an imbalance in your gut health.

What Are the Common Signs of Food Intolerance?

As mentioned above, the signs of food intolerance vary from person to person. Some of the most common signs of food intolerance include bloating, stomach aches, diarrhea, gas, fatigue, headaches, and skin rashes. However, many people with food intolerance may not experience any of these symptoms, which is why it is important to be aware of other signs, too. You may have food intolerance if you notice that you have digestive issues such as bloating, gas, diarrhea, or constipation after eating a certain food. If a certain food makes you feel tired, moody, or have a headache, you might have food intolerance, too. Food intolerance can also affect your mental health and can cause anxiety, panic attacks, and depression. Food intolerance can also be a sign of an imbalance in your gut health.

How to Test for Food Intolerance?

There are many different ways you can test for food intolerance. You can get a blood test, a stool test, or an allergen patch test. Some doctors may also recommend an elimination diet, where you completely stop eating certain foods for a certain amount of time so that your body can detoxify and heal. Food intolerance can be controlled and often even resolved by following certain diets or taking certain supplements. You can test for food intolerance by following an elimination diet, where you completely stop eating certain foods for a certain amount of time. During this time, your body will have time to heal and detoxify, which means you will see and know if a certain food is causing an adverse reaction. You can also get a blood test to test for food intolerance. However, it is important to know that blood tests for food intolerance are not always accurate.

The Link Between Food Intolerance and Gut Health

Food intolerance not only affects the way your body processes certain foods, but also the way your gut health functions. If you have food intolerance, it means that your gut isn't able to fully process certain foods properly. This can lead to an upset balance in your gut health, which can cause issues like bloating, constipation, diarrhea, and SIBO (small intestinal bacterial overgrowth). These issues can then lead to a variety of health issues. For example, undiagnosed food intolerance can lead to issues like low energy, depression, and anxiety, as well as increased risk of heart disease and stroke. Food intolerance can also cause damage to your gut health and can lead to various digestive issues.

Tips to Help Manage Food Intolerance and Gut Health

If you have food intolerance, you need to follow certain dietary restrictions. The first step to managing food intolerance is taking note of the symptoms you have after eating certain foods. It is important to note how long the symptoms last and how bad they are. By taking note of these symptoms, you can start to make connections between foods you eat and your reactions. Next, you should start to take control of your diet. Avoid eating the foods that you know cause adverse reactions in your body. However, you don't have to completely eliminate the foods that cause adverse reactions in you. Instead, you can substitute them with healthier alternatives. For example, if you have a milk intolerance, you can still have yogurt or cheese, but you can substitute milk in your coffee with almond milk, or if you have a gluten intolerance, you can still eat bread, but you can substitute gluten-containing flour with gluten-free flour. It is important to remember that even though food intolerance can cause issues, it is not an autoimmune disease. It can be managed by following certain dietary restrictions, but it does not need to be treated with the same attention as autoimmune diseases do.

Food intolerance can be a nuisance, with some people experiencing more serious symptoms than others. However, it is important to know that it is not something you need to worry about too much, and that there are many effective treatments and management strategies for it. If you believe that you have food intolerance, you can test for it by taking note of the symptoms you have after eating certain foods, and substituting them with healthier alternatives. With that in mind, you can take steps to prevent or manage any complications of food intolerance, including issues with gut health. With proper management, you can take advantage of the many benefits that come with food intolerance, such as improved health and energy, and a lowered risk of developing heart disease and stroke.

CHAPTER 6
GUT HEALTH FOR
PREGNANT WOMEN

During pregnancy, you may notice changes in your body. You may feel tired, bloated, or experience other symptoms. These are normal during pregnancy, however, if these symptoms become severe, you should contact your doctor immediately. This section will discuss what causes these symptoms and ways to improve gut health during pregnancy.

The Importance of Gut Health During Pregnancy

Gut health is of paramount importance during pregnancy since it helps to improve the health of the mother and the foetus. This section looks at the importance of gut health, as well as the changes that take place in the gut during pregnancy, and how to improve gut health. The digestive tract is made up of the stomach, small intestine, colon, and rectum. The colon and rectum are involved in defecation, whereas the small intestine is involved in the absorption of nutrients from the food that we eat. The small intestine also acts as a barrier that separates the body from its external environment. When we speak of gut health, we are referring to the health of the entire digestive tract, not just the small intestine. We will now take a brief look at the importance of gut health during pregnancy, as well as the changes that take place in the gut during pregnancy, and ways to improve gut health.

Gut health during pregnancy

Gut health is very important during pregnancy, as it helps to improve immune function, supports the health of the uterus, and helps to prevent constipation. During pregnancy, your gastrointestinal tract is stretched to its maximum length, and the hormones that are released by your body also change. This can increase the risk of certain health issues, so it's especially important to keep it healthy during this time. A healthy digestive tract can help to prevent morning sickness, avoid constipation, and support the growth of the unborn baby. The best way to keep your gut healthy during pregnancy is by following a diet that is high in fibre, contains plenty of fluids, and is low in fat and sugar. Another important thing to remember is that you should avoid eating before bedtime, since it can increase the risk of constipation. You should also avoid eating acidic foods, since they can increase acidity in your stomach. Most pregnant women find that they get constipation, so it's important to drink plenty of fluids and try not to eat too much fibre, which can make it worse.

Importance of diet during pregnancy

The type of foods that you eat during pregnancy can have a big impact on the health of both you and your baby. There are many reasons why improving gut health is so important during pregnancy, including that: - Your diet can help to prevent morning sickness, which can be a regular symptom during this time. - You can benefit from the extra nutrients that come from eating a healthy diet, such as fibre, vitamins, minerals, and proteins. - The foods that you eat have a direct impact on your immune system, so you can improve gut health and support your immune system during pregnancy.

Changes that take place in the gut during pregnancy

During pregnancy, there are many changes that take place in the gut, including an increase in the amount of blood that is delivered to the intestine and an increase in the amount of mucus produced by the gut. These changes are designed to increase the strength of the gut barrier that protects the body from the outside environment, and help to prevent bacteria from entering the body. The most important change that occurs in the gut is an increase in the amount of Bifidobacteria and Lactobacillus in pregnant women. This increase helps to prevent constipation, supports the growth of the unborn baby, and prevents an unhealthy metabolic balance in the mother. You can also benefit from improved gut motility during pregnancy. This is when the gut muscles contract and relax at the right time during digestion, which allows food to be absorbed properly.

Ways to improve gut health during pregnancy

The most important thing that you can do to improve gut health during pregnancy is to eat a diet high in fibre, which is low in fat, sugar, and sodium. You can also eat foods that are high in probiotics, such as yogurt and kefir. You can also take a probiotic supplement during pregnancy to help to boost the beneficial bacteria in your gut. A healthy diet is the best way to improve gut health during pregnancy, but there are also other things that you can do.

Ways to harm gut health during pregnancy

Eating too much fat and sugar can harm gut health during pregnancy, so it is important to keep your diet nutritious. You can also harm your gut health by consuming too much alcohol or caffeine. You should also try to avoid unhealthy foods, as well as taking medications that can harm the digestive tract. When you take medications, it is important to follow the directions for taking them, as well as to avoid taking any others that can harm your gut. You should also avoid overexerting yourself, as this can harm gut health.

How your gut health affects your unborn baby

The health of your digestive tract can affect the health of your unborn baby. This is because babies start to build their gut bacteria right after birth. If your digestive tract is unhealthy, then this could cause problems for your baby. Some of the factors that can affect your gut health and the health of your unborn baby include: - Your diet during pregnancy - This can affect the type of bacteria that are present in your gut. - Your fitness level - This can affect the amount of air that your gut gets, which is important for the development of your gut bacteria. - Your stress level - This can affect your nervous system and the health of your gut. - Your genetics - This can affect the health of your gut bacteria.

During pregnancy, your digestive tract is stretched to its maximum length and this can increase the risk of certain health issues. A healthy digestive tract can help to prevent morning sickness, avoid constipation, and support the growth of the unborn baby. You can improve gut health by following a diet that is high in fibre, contains plenty of fluids, and is low in fat and sugar. You can also take a probiotic supplement to help to boost the beneficial bacteria in your gut.

Gut Health Myths That All Pregnant Women Should Avoid

It can be hard to know what to believe about your gut and its health. With so much conflicting advice about everything from probiotics to artificial sweeteners, it can be difficult to know which "gut-friendly" advice is worth listening to. That's why you'll find this section on the topic of gut health packed with everything you need to know to keep your gut happy and healthy throughout your pregnancy. We will dispel the myths about your digestive system, as well as dispel some common concerns about gut health.

Proprietary Probiotics aren't helpful for gut health

Probiotic supplements are often advertised as a quick fix for digestive issues. After all, the logic goes, if you purchase probiotics and drink them, your gut should be improved immediately. But, the truth is, probiotics are effective only under specific conditions. In order to work, probiotics require that you: Be consuming a sufficient amount of water Be consuming a sufficient amount of prebiotic fibre Be eating an unhealthy diet that's lacking in bacteria These three factors are necessary for probiotics to be successful. If any one of them is missing, probiotics will have no effect on gut health.

Avoiding Meat won't help heal your gut

The idea that a gut full of "toxic" meat shouldn't be a healthy one. The fact is, the human gut is home to trillions of bacteria. And, while we do have bacteria in our gut that can be considered "pathogenic", we also have bacteria that are absolutely necessary to maintaining gut health. The gut is no place for toxic, harmful bacteria. So, why not try to heal your gut by adding more beneficial bacteria? One of the easiest ways to do this is by supplementing with probiotics!

Don't Avoid Antibiotics to help gut health

Antibiotics are often considered "bad" for gut health. But, the truth is, antibiotics can be a very beneficial part of a healthy pregnancy diet. Many pregnant women will avoid antibiotics due to the gut health myths above. But, before you start worrying about getting antibiotics and disrupting your gut's bacterial balance, let's take a closer look at how antibiotics are actually used during pregnancy. Current guidelines recommend that pregnant women can receive antibiotics in two situations: When a woman is in labour When a woman is breastfeeding For both of these situations, the benefits of antibiotic treatment far outweigh the risks associated with antibiotics.

Artificial Sweeteners won't affect gut health

Artificial sweeteners are commonly believed to be harmful to your gut. This is often due to the fact that low-calorie sweeteners aren't absorbed by the body. But, the truth is, artificial sweeteners can have a positive effect on gut health. First, it's important to note that artificial sweeteners aren't "unhealthy" by themselves. In fact, studies have found that the side effects of sweeteners like aspartame are minimal. Instead, the side effects of artificial sweeteners occur when they're consumed in large quantities. When consumed in moderation, however, artificial sweeteners like aspartame can actually help with digestion. One study found that consuming an artificially sweetened beverage after a meal could help to reduce the amount of food that you would otherwise feel hungry for.

Fermented foods may help your gut... or not

Fermented foods are often touted as a great way to "help your gut". Probiotic foods come in all shapes and forms, from probiotic yogurts to probiotic breads to probiotic pickles. But, the question is, are probiotic foods effective? And, if so, how? There are two factors that determine if fermented foods can improve gut health. The first is the probiotic bacteria that they contain. Probiotics must be able to survive the acidic environment of the stomach and make it past the small intestine intact. The second factor is the fermentation process used to "ferment" the foods. Fermentation must result in highly-absorbable vitamins and minerals.

Caffeine has no affect on gut health

It's often believed that caffeine can be a problem for gut health. After all, isn't caffeine a "drug"? But, here's the thing. Not all sources of caffeine are created equal. While some sources of caffeine are "drugs", others are perfectly natural. One of the most commonly-consumed sources of caffeine is coffee. Coffee contains caffeine, but it also contains a rich array of antioxidants and minerals. This means that coffee could actually be good for gut health! This is especially true if you're pregnant or breastfeeding. Studies have found that women who consume caffeine have a lower risk of developing gestational diabetes.

Artificial Sweeteners don't affect gut health

Artificial sweeteners are commonly believed to be harmful to your gut. This is often due to the fact that low-calorie sweeteners aren't absorbed by the body. But, the truth is, artificial sweeteners can have a positive effect on gut health. First, it's important to note that artificial sweeteners aren't "unhealthy" by themselves. In fact, studies have found that the side effects of sweeteners like aspartame are minimal. Instead, the side effects of artificial sweeteners occur when they're consumed in large quantities. When consumed in moderation, however, artificial sweeteners can actually help with digestion. One study found that consuming an artificially sweetened beverage after a meal could help to reduce the amount of food that you would otherwise feel hungry for.

Don't avoid Artificial colourings

Artificial colourings are often thought to be dangerous to your gut health. However, no evidence has been found to support this idea. In fact, artificial colourings actually have a number of benefits. In order to be effective, artificial colouring must be made up of certain compounds called carotenoids. These compounds provide many different health benefits. For example, one type of carotenoid known as beta-carotene helps boost immune function. Another type of carotenoids called lycopene helps protect against cancer. So, while there haven't been any reports of negative effects, it's still best to stay away from processed foods that use artificial colours.

How to Maintain a Healthy Gut During Pregnancy

Pregnancy is a time of tremendous change for your body and your diet. As you grow an additional person, your body undergoes rapid changes in preparation for baby. Changes in the digestive tract are among the most dramatic. Your digestive system undergoes a shift from processing small meals several times a day to taking in larger amounts of food at once and digesting it slowly over the course of days and weeks. This change is necessary to meet the increased energy requirements of pregnancy, but it can sometimes come at the expense of your digestive health. Luckily, you can keep your digestive system in tip-top shape while pregnant by following a few simple maintenance tips. A healthy gut is essential for your digestion and your overall wellbeing. A stable, functioning gut promotes regular bowel movements and helps prevent diarrhea, constipation, and other digestive issues. It also helps your body absorb nutrients from food. But sustaining a healthy gut doesn't just benefit you; your baby will also reap the benefits too. A healthy digestive system protects against eczema, colic, and other allergies. And, as you know from the change your digestive system experiences during pregnancy, a healthy gut is also essential for a smooth delivery.

Eat green and whole foods

Although you may have heard that you shouldn't eat fruits or vegetables during pregnancy because they may not be digested properly and could pose a risk to your health, you should eat plenty of green and orange vegetables and whole fruits. These are all healthy foods that are digested just fine during pregnancy. Fruits and vegetables can provide you with vitamins and minerals that your body needs for healthy growth, and whole fruits and vegetables are digested slowly, so you have time to digest them. When you eat vegetables that are green and leafy, you're not only getting more vitamins and minerals from a single serving, you're also getting fibre - the good type of fibre, not the type that can cause constipation. And fibre is essential for regular bowel movements, which can help prevent constipation, a common pregnancy problem.

Eat good fats

A healthy diet should include a balance of protein, carbohydrates, and fat. During pregnancy, your body needs more energy than usual, so you need to eat foods that provide it. Protein, carbohydrate and fat are all types of nutrients that your body uses to promote healthy growth and development. The best way to ensure you're eating a healthy diet during pregnancy is to eat a balanced amount of all three. Foods rich in good fats include oils such as olive, coconut, and flaxseed oil, avocados, nuts, and fish. Fats are stored energy, so you don't need to eat excess amounts, and they're also digested with ease by your body during pregnancy.

Eat fermented foods

During pregnancy, your digestive system undergoes a rapid change. Your stomach expands and your intestines undergo significant growth. This means that you need to eat more fibre and probiotics - bacteria that are essential for digestive health - than usual. Studies have found that consuming probiotics in fermented foods like yogurt, kefir, sauerkraut, and kimchi has been shown to improve gut health in women during pregnancy.

Make sure you're getting enough fiber

During pregnancy, your digestive system requires more fibre than usual. While all fruits and vegetables provide fibre, not all foods are high in fibre. Make sure that the foods you eat are "whole grains" such as whole wheat bread, brown rice, and quinoa. Whole grains are digested slowly, so you have time to digest your meals. They contain fiber, vitamins, minerals and other nutrients your body needs. They can also reduce your risk of heart disease, diabetes, and certain cancers.

Don't overeat starch

Starch is a type of carbohydrate that provides energy. During pregnancy, your body needs more energy than usual, so you need to eat foods that provide it. Foods high in starch include whole grains, potatoes, corn, and rice. But don't overdo it! Too much starch can lead to increased insulin production, which is why it's important to keep your carb intake moderate. You don't need to cut out carbs completely; you just need to keep your carb intake moderate. Moderate carb intake during pregnancy is when you eat them with protein or fat and not alone. Starchy foods should make up less than 30% of your daily calories.

Drink plenty of water

You may have heard that water should be avoided during pregnancy because it doesn't hydrate your body. This isn't true - in fact, staying hydrated is imperative to your health, especially during pregnancy. During pregnancy, your blood volume increases by about 30%, and this can lead to dehydration. One way to combat dehydration is by drinking plenty of water. Water helps your body function normally by regulating your digestive system, regulating your hormone levels, and promoting healthy skin. During pregnancy, your body needs more energy than usual, so you need to eat foods that provide it. Foods high in starch include whole grains, potatoes, corn, and rice. But don't overdo it! Too much starch can lead to increased insulin production, which is why it's important to keep your carb intake moderate. You don't need to cut out carbs completely; you just need to keep your carb intake moderate. Moderate carb intake during pregnancy is when you eat them with protein or fat and not alone. Starchy foods should make up less than 30% of your daily calories.

Eat a Balanced Diet

During pregnancy, your digestive system requires more energy than usual. This is why a balanced diet that includes protein, carbs, and good fats is so important. Protein, carb, and fat are all nutrients your body needs to promote healthy growth and development. A balanced diet can help you maintain a healthy gut. It can also help you feel better and be more active during pregnancy. A healthy pregnancy diet should include: - Plenty of vegetables - A variety of colours and textures are good for you, so try to eat as many as possible. - A source of protein - Protein helps build and repair your body after the growing that occurs during pregnancy. Choose lean sources of protein, such as fish, poultry, beans, soy products, and eggs. - Plenty of fruits - Fruits are rich in vitamins and minerals, which are essential for good health. - Moderate amounts of whole grains - Whole grains are a type of carbohydrate that provides energy. - A small amount of dairy products - If you can tolerate dairy during pregnancy, choose low-fat or fat-free milk, yogurt, and cheese.

Ditch the processed foods

During pregnancy, your body needs more energy than usual, so you need to eat foods that provide it. Foods high in sugar and processed grains are not digested well during pregnancy and are quickly converted into glucose, a type of carbohydrate your body needs but can't make itself. These foods can damage your digestive system and promote weight gain. The best thing you can do for your gut health during pregnancy is to ditch the processed foods from your diet. These foods are high in sugar, salt, and processed ingredients that won't provide you with the nutrients your body needs. Examples include white bread, pastries, sugary beverages, chips, and French fries. While these foods may taste delicious, they aren't good for your gut and may promote weight gain and create a risk for developing diabetes.

Decrease stress

Stress is a normal part of life, but it can be harmful when it's prolonged or chronic. During pregnancy, you need to protect your body from the physical and emotional damage that stress can cause. Maintaining a healthy emotional state by avoiding prolonged stress is essential for the well-being of both you and your baby. You can reduce stress by finding ways to relax throughout the day. Try taking a short walk outside, listening to music, meditating, doing yoga poses, reading, or watching television. Avoiding stressful situations altogether is another great way to manage stress. When dealing with a stressful situation, take deep breaths and remind yourself that you will be okay.

Get enough sleep

Sleep plays an important role in maintaining your overall wellbeing. Lack of sleep can negatively affect your mood, appetite, and general quality of life. In addition, lack of sleep has been linked to several complications during pregnancy including gestational diabetes, preterm labour, and miscarriage. Make sure you get at least eight hours of sleep per night.

If you're pregnant, you should definitely take steps to maintain a healthy gut during pregnancy. This includes eating foods rich in probiotics (like yogurt) and prebiotic fibers (like garlic), taking probiotic supplements, and avoiding antibiotics. But even if you aren't pregnant, it's still worth doing. Your gut plays a huge role in your overall health, and when it's unhealthy, it can affect everything from your moods to your skin to your ability to lose weight. So, eat well, exercise regularly, and pay attention to your gut—you'll feel better, look better, and have a healthier baby!

CHAPTER 7
GUT HEALTH FOR BREASTFEEDING MOTHERS

BREASTFEEDING IS great for both mom and baby, but sometimes moms get sick during pregnancy and may not feel well enough to breastfeed.

When you're pregnant, you should try to stay healthy as possible. This means eating nutritious foods, drinking lots of water, and taking care of yourself mentally and physically.

When you're breastfeeding, you should also do everything you can to make sure you stay healthy. In fact, breastfeeding moms who take care of themselves while pregnant will have healthier babies and toddlers.

In this chapter I'll tell you how to stay healthy during pregnancy and breastfeeding. I'll also share with you the top things every mother needs to do to ensure her optimal gut health and the best health of the child.

Why Maintaining Gut Health is Important for Breastfeeding Mothers

Breastfeeding is one of the most natural things a mother can do. The act of feeding your baby is what makes them a part of your family. When your baby latches on to your breast for the first time, a bond is formed that will last a lifetime. This is why many new mums choose to breastfeed their babies. If you choose to breastfeed, you want to make sure that you keep your baby healthy. For the mother, it is a demanding task. It is also beneficial to the baby. The benefits of breastfeeding are numerous. You can only achieve this if you have a healthy gut. This is why maintaining your gut health while breastfeeding is so important.

Gut health and breastfeeding

Many new mums have the misconception that breastfeeding is enough to keep their babies gut healthy. This, of course, is not the case. Breastmilk is only one source of nutrients for your baby. To stay healthy, both the mother and the baby must have the right diet. As breastfeeding is a natural process, it is no wonder that some mothers may experience digestive issues. If this happens to you, you are not alone. The majority of breastfeeding mums struggle with some kind of digestive problem. These issues occur mainly because of the lack of good gut flora in the mothers' system. By maintaining your gut health, you can prevent these issues from occurring.

You Are What You Eat

During your pregnancy you should focus on eating the right foods for both of you. Your infant will be nourished by the nutrients from your diet. You should maintain a healthy diet during breastfeeding as well. This way, you will have the right amount of energy to meet the needs of your baby. Foods rich in fibre and vitamins will help you stay healthy. Fibre will help you stay regular, while vitamins will help you avoid deficiencies. Some examples of fibre-rich foods are whole wheat bread, whole grain cereals, brown rice, oatmeal, and bran flakes.

Gut Flora Is KEY

The bacteria in your gut arc what make you healthy. A healthy gut flora is important to your overall health. A healthy gut flora is what helps you digest your food properly and stay regular. When you are not properly nourished, your gut flora will be disrupted. You will experience digestive issues, such as constipation, diarrhea, and bloating. If you are not experiencing any of these issues, there is a high chance that your gut flora is off. You can feed your gut flora by eating probiotic-rich foods.

Helps protect baby from infections

Breastmilk is one of the best sources of nutrition for your baby. It is full of antibodies, which protect your baby from infections. This is why the World Health Organization has recommended breastfeeding for over two years. It is the only food that has all of the essential nutrients your child needs. When your gut health is not optimal, your baby will not get the same benefits from breastfeeding. This is why maintaining your gut health while breastfeeding is so important.

Nutrients the baby gets

Breastmilk is a perfect source of nutrition for your baby. Although it is similar to human milk, it is different in many ways. One of the differences is the amount of nutrients it has. Breastmilk is composed of different proteins, carbohydrates, electrolytes, vitamins, and minerals. Breastmilk is the most complete food for your baby. Because it contains everything your child needs, it is the perfect food for them. It is also the most efficient food for feeding your baby.

Proven Benefits of breastfeeding

Breastfeeding can do so much for your baby. It is one of the most natural things a mother can do. It has been proven that babies who are breastfed are less likely to develop asthma, allergies, and obesity. Breastmilk has antibodies, which protect your child from infections. It also contains pre-digestive enzymes, which help your baby digest food easily. This will help your baby grow faster, smarter, and healthier. Breastfeeding also gives you a feeling of bonding with your baby. You will feel closer to your child after breastfeeding for a few months.

Gut Health and Breastmilk

During pregnancy, the mother's gut health is extremely important. Unfortunately, many women experience derailed gut health during pregnancy; however, when they breastfeed, the gut health typically returns to normal. During breastfeeding, your gut health is directly related to the quality and quantity of the milk your woman produces. If your gut health is not optimal, your milk will also be of poor quality and quantity. It is important to note that the bacteria in your gut, as well as the enzymes in your saliva, are passed down to your baby through your milk. Therefore, it is important to maintain your gut health while breastfeeding.

Maintaining Gut Health while Breastfeeding

There are many ways to keep your gut health strong while breastfeeding. One of the most effective ways is to eat probiotic-rich foods. Probiotic-rich foods are ideal for gut health because they contain beneficial bacteria. Some examples of probiotic-rich foods are yogurt, kefir, sauerkraut, kimchi, and pickles. Probiotic-rich foods will help your body fight off harmful bacteria and viruses. This will help you stay healthy and protect your baby from infections. You should also drink lots of water when you are breastfeeding. Water is necessary for digestion, so it is important for you to stay hydrated.

Lastly, you should make sure to get plenty of rest every day. When you are well rested, your body will be able to heal more quickly.

Breastfeeding is one of the most natural things a mother can do. The act of feeding your baby is what makes them a part of your family. When your baby latches on to your breast for the first time, a bond is formed that will last a lifetime. This is why many new mots choose to breastfeed their babies. If you choose to breastfeed, you want to make sure that you keep your baby healthy. For the mother, it is a demanding task. It is also beneficial to the baby. The benefits of breastfeeding are numerous. You can only achieve this if you have a healthy gut. This is why maintaining your gut health while breastfeeding is so important.

Tips to Keep Your Gut Healthy for Breastfeeding Mothers

Did you know that your digestive system has a direct impact on your breast milk? Your gut is home to trillions of microorganisms called microbiota, which play a vital role in your health. When you have a healthy and balanced gut, you tend to produce the best-quality breast milk. And yes, even the healthiest of diets can't guarantee you'll have the best quality breast milk. So yes, keeping your gut healthy for breastfeeding mothers isn't just a slogan. It's a necessity for producing the best-quality breast milk. You see, your breast milk is a perfect balance of fatty acids, amino acids, vitamins, minerals, enzymes, hormones, and other compounds. However, when you have a gut imbalance, you don't have the required bacteria and nutrients to produce breast milk. To have the best-quality breast milk, you need to feed your gut with the right foods, which is exactly what you'll learn about in this section.

What Is a Bifidobacteria Gut?

A bifidobacteria gut is the healthy ecosystem in your digestive system that contains bacteria that are beneficial to your health. Bifidobacteria is a type of bacteria that can be found in the human gut. Your gut bacteria change from person to person, and it's usually a healthy, diverse ecosystem that has a major impact on your health. Bifidobacteria are usually found in the human gut. Bifidobacteria are usually found in the human gut. The human gut has a complex ecosystem of bacteria. While many of these bacteria are present in all of us, some are present in very low levels and are called "neglected" bacteria. Bifidobacteria are usually found in the human gut. Bifidobacteria are usually found in the human gut. Bifidobacteria are usually found in the human gut. Bifidobacteria are usually found in the human gut.

What Is an Overgrowth of Bacteria?

When you have too much of a certain type of bacteria, this is called an overgrowth of the bacteria. Overgrowth of bacteria can occur when you have a weak immune system, a diet low in fiber and whole grains, or don't drink enough water. A healthy gut is supposed to be a very low bacterial count, and when it's too high, this can impact your health. Overgrowth of bacteria can occur when you have a weak immune system, a diet low in fiber and whole grains, or don't drink enough water. A healthy gut is supposed to be a very low bacterial count, and when it's too high, this can impact your health. Overgrowth of bacteria can occur when you have a weak immune system, a diet low in fiber and whole grains, or don't drink enough water. A healthy gut is supposed to be a very low bacterial count, and when it's too high, this can impact your health. Overgrowth of bacteria can occur when you have a weak immune system, a diet low in fiber and whole grains, or don't drink enough water. A healthy gut is supposed to be a very low bacterial count, and when it's too high, this can impact your health. Overgrowth of bacteria can occur when you have a weak immune system, a diet low in fiber and whole grains, or don't drink enough water. A healthy gut is supposed to be a very low bacterial count, and when it's too high, this can impact your health. Overgrowth of bacteria can occur when you have a weak immune system, a diet low in fiber and whole grains, or don't drink enough water. A healthy gut is supposed to be a very low bacterial count, and when it's too high, this can impact your health. Overgrowth of bacteria can occur when you have a weak immune system, a diet low in fiber and whole grains, or don't drink enough water. A healthy gut is supposed to be a very low bacterial count, and when it's too high, this can impact your health.

Drink Enough Water

This is a no-brainer, right? If you don't drink enough water, your gut will be in trouble. Your gut is actually made up of around 70% water, so you can imagine how important it is to hydrate your gut. Water is essential for your gut's bacterial balance and helps to keep your digestive system working optimally. Keep in mind that water is not just for your body – it is also for your gut. As we discussed above, your gut is about 70% water. Without enough water, the good bacteria in your gut are not able to grow. And that's not good for your health. Water is essential for your gut's bacterial balance and helps to keep your digestive system working optimally.

Avoid Processed Foods

Many processed foods are full of sugar and preservatives, which can wreak havoc on your digestive system. And yes, even if the label says "no sugar added," sugar is sugar. It doesn't matter if it's in a pill, a fruit juice, a ketchup, or a cake – too much sugar will negatively impact your gut health. So how can you tell if a food is processed? When you read the ingredient list of foods, look for words like "hydrogenated," "high fructose corn syrup," "sugar," "funky corn starch," "artificial flavoring," "artificial preservatives," "artificial colors," and "high salt."

Stay Active

You can't out-exercise bad diet, so make sure you're eating a healthy, balanced diet. And one of the best ways to stay active is to walk! Studies suggest that walking is the perfect exercise for gut health. It increases your metabolic rate (the number of calories you burn while resting), it strengthens your digestive system, and it reduces your appetite. Walking is a great exercise for gut health. Walking is a great exercise for gut health.

Avoid Smoking

Smoking is a major cause of poor gut health, and it can lead to a number of health problems. Smoking is harmful to your gut bacteria, which are necessary for a healthy digestive system. Additionally, smoking can lead to an overgrowth of harmful bacteria in your gut, which can lead to digestive issues and even an overgrowth of bacteria.

Keep your Home Clean

How clean is clean? You want your home to be as clean as your body. You want to avoid anything that might affect your gut bacteria, such as household cleaning products that contain alcohol or bleach, harsh household cleaners, and dirty surfaces. These things can damage your gut bacteria and make it harder for you to digest food properly.

Get Enough Good Bacteria

You can't feed your gut with bad bacteria – it's just not going to work. Your gut needs beneficial bacteria to function properly. The healthiest way to feed your gut with good bacteria is to feed your probiotic with probiotic yogurt. Probiotic yogurt contains live bacteria and works pretty well to keep your gut healthy and strong. You can also feed your probiotics with probiotic supplements, which are easier to take than a yogurt.

Don't Drink Alcohol

Boozy beverages are terrible for your gut health. Alcohol is inflammatory and can lead to an imbalance of gut bacteria, which can ultimately harm your digestive system. While moderate alcohol consumption is fine for most people, pregnant women and breast-feeding mothers should avoid alcohol completely. Excessive drinking can lead to an overgrowth of harmful bacteria in your gut, which can lead to digestive issues, such as constipation, diarrhea, and bloating.

Alkaline Diet

The acidity in your stomach is crucial for your gut health. When your stomach is too acidic, it can damage your digestive system and lead to an overgrowth of harmful bacteria. The acidity in your stomach is crucial for your gut health. When your stomach is too acidic, it can damage your digestive system and lead to an overgrowth of harmful bacteria. The best way to reduce your stomach acidity is to consume an alkaline diet. Alkaline diets are based on the idea that eating too many acidic foods, such as fruits, vegetables, and dairy products, can lead to an overly acidic stomach. Therefore, an alkaline diet is designed to help balance your stomach pH levels. This helps to prevent an overgrowth of harmful microbes and keeps your digestive system functioning properly.

Probiotic Supplements to Balance Your Gut During Breastfeeding

The benefits of probiotic supplementation during pregnancy and lactation have been recognized by researchers around the world since the 1990s. In fact, most doctors recommend supplementing with probiotics during these times because they know how important it is to maintain a healthy gut environment. However, did you know that there are significant differences between the types of probiotics used during pregnancy and lactation? Here we will discuss some of the key differences between them:

Probiotic Supplementation During Pregnancy

While probiotic supplementation has become increasingly popular among pregnant and breastfeeding moms, its effectiveness remains somewhat controversial. Some studies suggest that probiotics may improve certain baby outcomes, but others say that there isn't enough evidence to support this claim. For example, one study found that taking probiotics was linked to higher rates of preterm birth (less than 37 weeks gestation) among babies born to mothers who were given the probiotic Lactobacillus rhamnosus GG. Another study showed that infants who received probiotics had lower rates of hospitalization and antibiotic use compared to those who didn't receive any probiotics. On the other hand, another study found no difference in infant mortality or gastrointestinal infections when comparing groups of children who took probiotics versus those who didn'ts take probiotics during their first year of life.

Probiotic Supplementations During Breastfeeding

During breastfeeding, probiotics are particularly beneficial because they help promote the growth of good bacteria in your digestive tract. Studies show that probiotics help increase breast milk supply, boost immune function, and protect against gastrointestinal illnesses. Additionally, probiotics may also be able to treat urinary tract infections, allergies, eczema, asthma, and even diabetes.

CHAPTER 8
GUT HEALTH HACKS FOR POST-MENOPAUSAL WOMEN

MENOPAUSE IS a natural part of aging. However, many women experience symptoms such as hot flashes, mood swings, fatigue, and vaginal dryness. These symptoms can make everyday tasks difficult and even dangerous.

There are several reasons why menopause affects women differently. Some women experience these symptoms because of hormone imbalances while others suffer from a lack of estrogen. In either case, the solution is simple: get more estrogen!

The most common gut health problems that affect post-menopausal women are easy to fix with diet and lifestyle changes. This includes tips for improving digestion, reducing bloating, and preventing constipation.

How to Improve Your Post-Menopausal Gut Health

The end of your reproductive years can leave you feeling exhausted, lonely, and sad. But that doesn't mean you have to miss out on the other phases of your life, too. As you enter your post-reproductive years, you're likely to experience hormonal changes that affect your body, mind, and spirit. But these changes don't mean the end of the world. They're just another natural phase that you can embrace as you become more self-aware of your needs and what you want from your future. Reading up on the latest nutrition and fitness trends can be a fun way to keep your mind and body active. But when it comes to keeping your gut healthy and feeling energized, it's important to understand the information you're getting.

Make Sure Your Body Has Enough Omega-3s

While omega-3s are great for your heart, they are also important for your gut health. The lining of your gut is made up of a type of bacteria called the gut microbiota, which helps regulate your digestion, immune system, and mood. A recent study found that people who consumed higher amounts of omega-3s had a healthier microbiota. An easy way to increase your omega-3 intake is to eat fatty fish, such as salmon, sardines, and mackerel. You can also supplement your diet with krill oil.

Get Enough Probiotics to Balance Your Bacteria

Probiotics are "good" bacteria that can be taken as a dietary supplement or consumed in fermented foods. Our microbiota can differ from person to person, which can affect our metabolism and health. A probiotic's job is to create a healthy balance by increasing the amount of "good" bacteria in your gut. Probiotics can be taken as a dietary supplement or consumed in fermented foods. Some probiotic-rich foods are yogurt, kefir, miso, sauerkraut, and kimchi. If you're looking for a probiotic that's easier to take, try a supplement.

Try These Gut-Healthy Fruits and Veggies

Healthy fruits and veggies can provide you with prebiotics, fibrous carbohydrates that can improve your digestive health by increasing the growth of "good" bacteria in your gut. Some of the best prebiotic foods are artichokes, asparagus, celery, garlic, leeks, lettuce, onions, and ginger. Just remember, you don't have to suffer from a case of the Runts if you don't want to!

Eat Fermented Foods

Fermented foods are a great source of probiotics and prebiotics. They can help your gut by increasing the amount of "good" bacteria in your gut. Fermented foods are traditionally made by adding a specific culture to food, such as lacto-fermentation with dairy or yeasts with grains. Some fermented foods that are great for gut health are: Yogurt, kefir, and buttermilk

Add Probiotics to Your Diet

Take a probiotic supplement or eat probiotic-rich foods for gut health. Probiotics can be taken as a dietary supplement or consumed in fermented foods. Some probiotic-rich foods are: Yogurt, kefir, and buttermilk

Make it a Meal Swap Day

One of the easiest ways to improve your gut health is to swap out some of your meals for others that are healthier and more beneficial for your gut. Instead of a cheeseburger for dinner, try a grilled chicken breast with vegetables instead. Also, be mindful of what you're eating. When you eat the wrong foods, it can affect the bacteria in your gut and cause digestive discomfort.

Gut-Boosting Exercise

It's important to remember that while physical activity helps with gut health, it's also important to engage in activities that help with mental well-being as well. So while cardio is great for your heart and helps with your weight loss goals, it's also important to include mental exercises like mindfulness or visualization.

Prebiotics and gut health

A diet rich in prebiotics can improve your gut health by encouraging the growth of "good" bacteria in your gut. Foods high in prebiotics include: Fermented vegetables like sauerkraut, kimchi, and miso

Healthy Fats for improved gut health

Healthy fats are important for your heart and brain health because they can help curb your appetite and reduce your cravings for unhealthy foods. Healthy fats can be obtained by eating: Olive oil Avocado nuts

3 ways to balance your microbiota

- Eat a diet high in probiotics and fiber. Try to include a variety of probiotic-rich foods in your diet. Fermented vegetables like sauerkraut, kimchi, and miso should be a part of your daily diet. - If you're looking for a probiotic that's easier to take, try a supplement. - Add probiotics to your diet by consuming probiotic-rich foods like yogurt, kefir, and fermented vegetables like sauerkraut, kimchi, and miso. - Get your heart pumping by doing cardiovascular activity like running, walking, cycling, etc.

CHAPTER 9
WHY VEGETARIAN WOMEN CAN HAVE GUT ISSUES AND WHAT TO DO ABOUT IT

VEGETARIAN DIETS CAN BE some of the most challenging for a woman's digestive system. Not only do they lack the essential nutrients found in animal-based foods, but they can also be devoid of key enzymes found in animal-based foods. This lack of enzymes, known as the lectin theory, is what causes problems in the digestive tract. To put it simply, plant-based foods lack the enzymes that are necessary to break down and assimilate nutrients in the same way that animal-based foods do. That being said, there are still likely to be other challenges for a vegetarian woman's digestive system that are specific to her and are not shared by all other vegans or vegetarians. As a result, veggie women may experience different symptoms than their carnivore counterparts, even if they follow the exact same diet. Cost of being a vegetarian: The first gut-check

What's in a Vegetarian Diet?

Vegetarian diets can be as simple or as complex as one desires. Some vegetarians may eat only white rice, while others may include cereal, pasta, legumes, rice, bread, and dairy as staples of their diets. The most important element of a vegetarian diet is the inclusion of plants as the main source of energy in the body. Vegetarians tend to eat more plant-based whole foods than they do animal-based foods, which is why they receive more fiber than omnivores. Plant fiber is important for digestive health since it helps to promote regularity and a healthy gut. Not only do fiber-rich foods fill you up, they also act as a "normalizer" for your digestive system.

How Does a Vegetarian Diet Affect the Body?

Vegetarians tend to have lower intakes of saturated fat, cholesterol, and sodium, meaning that they tend to be healthier than non-vegetarians. This can be attributed to the fact that vegetarian diets tend to be lower in calories (and thus lower in fat) and higher in fiber, two things that can contribute to weight loss. Still, vegetarians often have to be mindful about how much they eat to avoid becoming too underweight or overweight. Vegetarians also may have lower intakes of iron and zinc, two minerals that are important for health and that are often limited in vegetarians due to lack of animal products. Vegetarian women may also have lower intakes of calcium, iron, zinc, and omega-3 fatty acids and higher intakes of copper and protein. However, there is no consistent evidence that one type of vegetarian diet is healthier than another in terms of nutrient intake.

What's the Difference Between a Vegan and Vegetarian Gut?

Vegetarians, who eat plant-based foods, may experience a reduced gut flora, while vegans, who eat no animal products at all, may experience an overgrowth of bacteria in the gut. The lectin theory, which describes the lack of enzymes in plant-based foods, is the explanation for both of these gut issues. It is important to note, however, that these issues are not unique to vegetarians; they are also experienced by non-vegetarians and occur for many different reasons. Both vegetarians and vegans have a reduced diversity of bacteria in the gut, meaning that the good bacteria that keep us healthy are likely missing. When this happens, the body may have an unusually high number of bad bacteria in the gut, which can lead to digestive issues and even an overgrowth of yeast or fungus in the gut. A healthy gut flora is important for digesting food, absorbing nutrients from food, and avoiding diseases. A key question to ask yourself is whether the changes you are experiencing are due to the amount of fiber or fruits and vegetables that you are eating. If these changes are occurring regardless of your diet, then it's likely that a healthy vegetarian diet is not the problem.

What causes gut issues for vegetarian women?

When you don't eat animal products, the nutrients that are typically found in animal products are missing from your diet, leaving your digestive system to work harder to break down and assimilate nutrients. Not only is this taxing on your digestive system, but it is also likely to lead to digestive system disruption. Research conducted in vegetarians and vegans suggests that the lack of essential nutrients (such as calcium, iron, zinc, and omega-3 fatty acids) and the lack of enzymes in plant-based foods may lead to digestive issues. These issues may be more prominent in vegetarian women because of their different nutritional needs. Vegetable-based diets may be low in iron, zinc, vitamin A, vitamin C, and other vitamins and minerals that may be important for vegans or vegetarians. They may also be low in calories and protein, which may contribute to underweight or malnourishment.

The Science Behind the Gut-Brain Connection

Scientists do not fully understand how the gut-brain connection works, but they do know that the gut plays a role in regulating mood, behavior, and stress. Ingesting fiber-rich foods, for example, may help to promote a sense of fullness, which may help to reduce anxiety and stress that are often associated with poor digestion and nutrient deficiencies. Low levels of serotonin in the gut have been linked to anxiety. Vitamin B6 and tryptophan found in Biotin (vitamin B7) may help to promote relaxation. Vitamin C, which is abundant in citrus fruits and vegetables, may help to promote a sense of calm.

Why Vegetarian Women Experience Issues with Their Gut?

Vegetarian diets do not provide the essential nutrients for the digestive system. As a result, vegetarians may experience deficiencies in the following areas: - Vitamin B - Vitamin B6 (pyridoxine) - Vitamin C - Calcium - Iron - Zinc Vegetarians may also experience poor digestion and nutrient deficiencies as a result of eating a diet devoid of animal products. As a result, vegetarians may require more fiber than omnivores to promote regularity and a healthy digestive system.

Why Vegetarian Women Can Have Gut Issues and What to Do About It

Vegetarian women may experience a reduced gut flora due to a lack of essential nutrients in their diet. These women can boost the levels of the following nutrients in their diets: - Vitamin B - Vitamin B6 - Vitamin C - Iron - Zinc Other gut issues that vegans and vegetarians may experience are bloating, constipation, cramps, and diarrhea. These issues are not specific to vegetarians and can also be experienced by non-vegetarians. There are a few key things to remember about maintaining a healthy digestive system. The first is to pay attention to your body. Notice how you feel after eating certain foods, how your bowel movements are progressing, and how you are feeling overall. The second is to make sure that you are getting enough sleep. Lastly, keep a journal and track your symptoms in order to better understand what may be causing them.

What Are the Different Challenges for a Vegetarian Woman's Gut?

Vegetarian diets are not designed to give your digestive tract what it needs to function optimally. That being said, a vegetarian diet can still have its challenges for a woman's digestive system based on what a vegetarian does eat. Vegetarians usually eat fewer calories than omnivores, which can make it harder to gain weight. Vegans and vegetarians also have fewer dietary cholesterol than omnivores to avoid, which can make it harder to maintain your weight. Vegans and vegetarians also live with a lower intake of vitamin B-12, iron, zinc, and other nutrients. The lack of certain nutrients can cause a lack of minerals in the body, which can lead to a variety of chronic conditions, including atherosclerosis and metabolic syndrome.

Strategies for a healthier digestive system

Give your gut flora the right "g-word." You can get probiotics in some drinks, yogurts, and as supplements. Make sure you drink lots of water and eat fibre-rich foods. Solve the calcium-water problem. If you have a hard time getting enough calcium in your diet, you can get it from a supplement. Try fermented foods. Fermented vegetables, such as sauerkraut, can be a great source of probiotics. You can also take a calcium supplement. Buy a high-powered blender and make your own veggie drinks. Try vegan diets. Vegan diets that include eggs, fish, and dairy can be very tasty and provide a lot of nutrients.

What to eat to feel better

Fibre - Vegetarians usually eat less fibre than omnivores, which can make it harder to feel satiated and full. Make sure you eat a lot of it, especially if you feel full too soon or not at all after eating. What's more, fibre can help you regulate your gut hormones, which can help you feel fuller longer. - Vegetarians usually eat less fibre than omnivores, which can make it harder to feel satiated and full. Make sure you eat a lot of it, especially if you feel full too soon or not at all after eating. What's more, fibre can help you regulate your gut hormones, which can help you feel fuller longer. Vitamin B-12 - Vegetarians usually get less vitamin B-12 than omnivores. Make sure you take a supplement. - Vegetarians usually get less vitamin B-12 than omnivores. Make sure you take a supplement. Iron - Vegans and vegetarians usually get less iron than omnivores. Make sure you take a supplement. - Veggans and vegetarians usually get less iron than omnivores. Make sure you take a supplement. Calcium - Vegans and vegetarians usually get less calcium than omnivores. You can try a vegan diet that includes dairy products, or take a supplement. - Veggans and vegetarians usually get less calcium than omnivores. You can try a vegan diet that includes dairy products, or take a supplement. Zinc - Vegans and vegetarians usually get less zinc than omnivores. Make sure you take a supplement. - Veggans and vegetarians usually get less zinc than omnivores. Make sure you take a supplement. Probiotics - Probiotics are "good" bacteria that can change your gut flora. Try fermented foods, or take probiotic supplements. - Probiotics are "good" bacteria that can change your gut flora. Try fermented foods, or take probiotic supplements. Water - You also need lots of water to function well. You can get more water by drinking half a gallon a day. Exercising - Exercising releases endorphins, which can make you feel better. What's more, doing so can increase your water intake by 10%.

CHAPTER 10
GUT HEALTH FOR VEGAN WOMEN: THE IMPORTANCE OF GUT MICROBIOME FOR VEGANS

You've probably heard about the importance of a healthy diet and regular exercise in maintaining a healthy life. However, did you know that a diet rich in fiber and probiotics is equally important for keeping your gut in check? In this chapter, we talk about the importance of a healthy gut for vegans and how our gut health can be improved by incorporating probiotics in our diets. We will explore what probiotics are, the connection between the gut and our immune system, the importance of a healthy gut microbiome, and the best foods for improving our gut health as a vegan.

What is a Gut Microbiome?

The gut microbiome is the collection of bacteria and viruses that live in our digestive system. It's estimated that we have over 500 different microorganisms living in our gut, and this diversity can be affected by diet, medication, and other factors. The majority of the microbes in our gut feed on food that our bodies produce, such as sugars, proteins, and vitamins. These microbes produce substances that our bodies can't produce on their own, such as vitamins, minerals, short-chain fatty acids, amino acids, and other compounds. Gut microbes also affect our immune system and our gastrointestinal health. Research has shown that a healthy gut microbiome is important for women's health.

Gut microbiome in vegan women

The gut microbiome has been studied in vegans and vegetarians, and some interesting findings were found. There were fewer bacterial species in the gut micro-biome of vegans than in people who eat animal prod-ucts, and the gut microbiome of vegans also contained fewer genes associated with protein digestion. The reason vegans might have a lower diversity of bacteria in their gut is not clear, but it's possible that the absence of animal proteins in vegan diets might induce a change in the gut microbiome. It's also possible that a lack of certain vitamins in a vegan diet could contribute to the change in the gut microbiome. Vegan women have reported that they have a harder time maintaining a healthy gut microbiome compared to non-vegan women. What's more, vegan women have also reported that they've had a lower libido and a lower quality of vaginal lubrication than non-vegan women.

The Connection Between the Gut and the Immune System

The gut is part of the immune system because it contains a large number of immune cells and immune system molecules, including immune molecules that are produced by our gut microbes. The process of breaking down complex dietary components into molecules that the body can use for energy, growth, and development is called digestion. The gut is where this process takes place. Not all of the molecules that are absorbed from the food you eat end up in the blood, which is the body's main transportation system. Some of the molecules that we eat are broken down by the cells in the gut, and part of these molecules get transported to other places in the body, such as the liver, muscles, bone tissue, fat tissue, and the brain. This process is called retransformation and it's important for our immune system. If a certain molecule is missing from the diet but is present in the gut, the gut microbes can retransform it so that it can be used by our immune system.

The Importance of a Healthy Gut Microbiome

A healthy gut microbiome is important for maintaining a healthy digestive system. A healthy gut microbiome is also important for your health and well-being, including your mood and sexual function. Many vegans report that they have a harder time maintaining a healthy gut microbiome than non-vegans do. One reason for this might be that, compared to omnivores, vegans have a diet that's less rich in fiber and probiotics. Vegan women have reported that they have a harder time maintaining a healthy gut microbiome than non-vegan women. This is likely because a vegan diet is rich in fiber and probiotics but is also missing some essential nutrients. Vegan women also have reported that they've had a lower libido and a lower quality of vaginal lubrication than non-vegan women. This is likely because a lack of some essential vitamins in a vegan diet can affect your vaginal health, which then may affect your libido.

The Best Foods for Improving Gut Health as a Vegan

The best foods for improving gut health as a vegan are those that are high in fiber and probiotics. Fiber is essential for gut health because it helps us to stay regular, it assists in the removal of toxins from the body, and it may even prevent certain diseases. High-fiber foods can be difficult to find in a vegan diet, so we recommend that you carry a food log to help you track your diet. Keeping a food log will help you to identify which foods are missing from your diet, and it will also help you to identify which foods you can add to your diet to improve your gut health. High-fiber foods include: - Whole-grain products like brown rice, whole-grain bread, whole-grain pasta, and whole-grain cereals - Fibrous vegetables like broccoli, cauliflower, and cabbage - Legumes like black beans, chickpeas, edamame, and lentils - Fruit like apples, oranges, and pears - Nuts like almonds, cashews, walnuts, and macadamias - Seeds like sesame, sunflower, and pumpkin

Tips for maintaining your gut microbiome as a vegan

- Maintain a high fiber diet. Fiber is best consumed at meals, and each meal should include a source of fiber. - Eat legumes with every meal. Legumes are rich in fibre, protein, and many vitamins and minerals that are beneficial to our health. - Drink plenty of water. Water is essential for the removal of toxins from our bodies and for regulating our pH levels. - Get plenty of sleep. We don't realize how important sleep is for maintaining a healthy gut health. - Don't stress out. Stress can affect your gut health by increasing your levels of cortisol, a hormone that can cause your digestive system to become more acidic. - Don't skip meals. Skipping meals can lead to low blood sugar, which can lead to an unhealthy increase in your levels of cortisol and an unhealthy decrease in your levels of glutathione, a molecule that helps to maintain the integrity of your digestive system.

The gut microbiome is important for vegans and vegetarians. The best foods for maintaining your gut microbiome as a vegan are those that are high in fiber and probiotics. Keeping your gut microbiome healthy is not only important for vegans, but for everyone who wants to stay healthy. Fiber is essential for your gut health, and probiotics are important for maintaining a healthy gut microbiome.

CHAPTER 11

HOW TO KEEP YOUR GUT HEALTH IN CHECK WHEN YOU'RE A GLUTEN-FREE WOMAN

FOR THOSE WHO might not know, gluten is a type of protein found in grains such as wheat and barley. It gives foods their chewy texture, as well as their distinctive taste. If you're a woman who's been diagnosed with celiac disease and aren't eating anything containing gluten, chances are you're probably missing out on whole grain foods and gluten-free alternatives. As a result, you'll probably have a negative impact on your gut health. However, this doesn't have to be the case. You can have your cake and eat it too, so to speak. In this article, we'll cover the top ways to keep your gut health in check when you're a gluten-free woman.

How gluten affects your gut health

The gut is responsible for absorbing nutrients from food so that they can be distributed throughout the rest of the body. This occurs via the tiny "villi" lining the gut. These villi are what we're interested in here, because they're how your gut receives nutrients. Unfortunately, when you consume gluten, the villi become "leaky" and start absorbing the gluten instead of nutrients. This leads to other health issues because it changes how the rest of the body absorbs nutrients. Other symptoms of gluten intolerance include bloating, diarrhea, constipation, and abdominal pain. As you can see, it's not just a "lazy" person's diet. If you're intolerant to gluten, you'll also have a weakened immune system, which can result in conditions such as leaky gut or celiac disease. This is why it's so important to keep your gut health in check.

Eat a Balanced Diet

The most important thing when it comes to keeping your gut health in check is eating a balanced diet. This means foods full of complex carbs, fiber, vitamins, minerals, and antioxidants. This is essential for maintaining a healthy gut. Unfortunately, many gluten-free diets are low in fiber, iron, and other nutrients. You can remedy this by adding more "whole foods" to your diet. Whole grains, legumes, vegetables, and fruits are all great sources of fiber. These foods keep your digestive system moving properly and make your gut happy. You can also eat foods rich in iron and vitamin B. Vitamin B can help reduce inflammation in the digestive system, which is why it's so important to keep your gut health in check.

Eat Fermented Foods

Fermented foods are a great way to get probiotics into your gut. Probiotics are the "good bacteria" in the gut. They're essential for your digestive health and even your immune system. To get the probiotics you need, you should eat a variety of fermented foods. This includes sauerkraut, kimchi, kefir, and yogurt. The good thing about fermented foods is that they're super simple to make at home. All you need are some basic ingredients and a jar. If you don't have time to make your own, you can easily buy it at the store. Another thing to keep in mind is to store them properly so they don't go bad. If you have time to pause, this is a good time to make a commitment to eat more fermented foods. They're packed with probiotics, which are essential for gut health.

Drink Fermented Beverages

You should also drink fermented beverages. This includes kombucha, cultured soy drink, and coconut water. Kombucha is a type of fermented tea and has a lot of health benefits. It can be a good source of probiotics and nutrients, and has even been proven to help with weight loss and gut health. Fermented soy drinks like tamari are also a good source of probiotics, and can be consumed as a replacement for soy sauce. Coconut water is a hydrating drink that's low in calories and high in electrolytes. These are essential minerals your body loses when you're dehydrated.

Take a Good Probiotic

If you're consuming a healthy diet full of fiber, probiotics, and fermented foods, then you should be good to go. However, if you're having trouble getting all of these nutrients into your system, then a probiotic supplement can help. There are tons of probiotics on the market, so it can be tricky to choose the right one for you. It's best to get the opinions of others and read reviews online. A probiotic supplement can be taken in liquid, capsule, or chewable form. Make sure you pick one that's high in probiotics, and that's also gentle on your gut. You can also combine probiotics with prebiotic foods, which are non-digestible foods that can "feed" the probiotics in your gut.

Don't Be Afraid of Fermented Foods

If you're eating a balanced diet, then there's no need to be afraid of fermented foods. In fact, they're great for you. Regardless of your diet, fermented foods can be a great source of probiotics. However, if you're gluten-free, this is especially true. The reason for this is because gluten is a type of protein found in grains that can negatively affect your gut health. When you consume gluten, the villi lining your gut become "leaky" and start absorbing the gluten instead of nutrients. This can lead to other health issues, like an imbalance in the digestive system and a weakened immune system. You can correct this by eating a balanced diet full of "whole foods" that provide fiber and other nutrients.

Exercise

Exercising is great for your health in just about every way possible. It can help you lose weight and prevent diabetes, for example. It can also help keep your gut health in check. This is because exercise helps you keep a healthy digestive system. This can be especially helpful for those on a gluten-free diet. Studies have shown that when people follow a gluten-free diet, their digestive systems become "leaky." To prevent this, you should exercise. This helps you keep the digestive system working properly, which is essential for your gut health. You can also try yoga, martial arts, and Pilates. These are all great ways to keep your gut health in check when you're gluten-free.

The most important thing when it comes to keeping your gut health in check is eating a balanced diet full of "whole foods." You can do this by including more fiber, vitamins, minerals, and probiotics into your diet. You can also drink fermented drinks, eat fermented foods, and exercise. The best way to do this is to make sure you're eating a balanced diet. This means foods full of complex carbs, fiber, vitamins, minerals, and antioxidants. You can also consume probiotics, which are essential for your gut health. Finally, exercise is great for keeping your gut health in check.

CHAPTER 12
GUT HEALTH RECIPES FOR WOMEN

YOUR DIGESTIVE SYSTEM is your body's largest organ. It's responsible for breaking down food and absorbing nutrients. Your digestive tract is made up of many different parts, including your stomach, small intestine, large intestine, pancreas, liver, gallbladder, spleen, appendix, colon, rectum, and anus.

There are many ways to improve your gut health, including eating healthy foods, getting regular exercise, and taking supplements. But there are also some natural remedies that can help you feel better and live longer.

Women need gut health just like men do. But unlike men, women tend to be more sensitive to foods that cause gas, bloating, and diarrhea. When you eat well, you feel better and live longer. So it makes sense that when you're looking for healthy recipes, you should be looking for recipes that support your gut health.

Here are some tips to help you find healthy recipes:

1. Look for recipes that include fiber. Fiber helps keep your digestion moving smoothly and supports regularity.

2. Avoid processed foods. Processed foods contain ingredients that aren't natural, like refined sugars, artificial sweeteners, preservatives, and additives. These ingredients disrupt the balance of bacteria in your gut.

3. Eat plenty of vegetables. Vegetables are packed with nutrients, including vitamins, minerals, antioxidants, and phytonutrients. They also contain fiber, which promotes regularity.

4. Choose whole grains over white flour. Whole grains are rich in fiber and protein, and they contain many beneficial compounds called phytochemicals.

5. Include beans, nuts, and seeds. Beans, nuts, and seeds are great sources of protein, fiber, and healthy fats. They also contain plant sterols, which may reduce cholesterol absorption.

6. Add probiotics. Probiotics are living microorganisms that help regulate the growth of other organisms in your gut.

Breakfast Recipes to Improve Gut Health

Gut health is very important for our body. We all know that our gut plays a vital role in our overall health. The food we eat has a direct impact on our gut health. In this section I am going to share with you some breakfast recipes that will help you to improve your gut health.

1. Banana Pancakes

Bananas are rich in potassium and fiber. They also contain vitamin B6, magnesium, folate, iron, zinc, copper, manganese, phosphorus, calcium, niacin, riboflavin, thiamine, pantothenic acid, and vitamins A and C. These ingredients are good for our digestive system.

Ingredients:

- 1 ripe banana

- 2 eggs

- ½ cup oatmeal

- ¼ teaspoon baking powder

- 1 tablespoon honey

- Milk as required

Preparation:

Preheat oven to 200 degrees Celsius (400 degrees Fahrenheit). Grease a non-stick frying pan with oil. Add bananas and cook until they turn golden brown. Remove from heat and let cool. Beat eggs well. Mix remaining ingredients together and add to egg mixture. Pour batter into greased frying pan and bake for 10 minutes. Flip pancakes over and bake for another 5 minutes. Serve hot.

Nutrition Information:

Calories: 190

Carbohydrates: 30 g

Protein: 9 g

Fat: 7 g

2. Oatmeal With Almonds And Honey

Oats are one of the best gluten free options available. They're high in fiber and low in fat. They have a mild flavor so they go well with most types of meals.

Almond meal is another option if you don't want to use oats. It contains magnesium, zinc, iron, calcium, phosphorus, and selenium, which are essential for bone development.

The combination of honey and almonds adds sweetness to the oatmeal. This recipe is perfect for breakfast or as an afternoon snack.

Ingredients:

½ cup rolled oats

¾ cup almond meal

⅓ cup honey

1 egg

1 teaspoon vanilla extract

Preparation: Combine all the ingredients in a bowl. Put the mixture into the oven at 350°F for about 20 minutes. You can serve the oatmeal hot or cold.

Nutrition Information

Calories: 230

Carbs: 38 g

Protein: 11 g

Fat: 8 g

3. Egg White Scramble

Egg whites are a good source of protein and they're easy to prepare. They also provide a lot of energy without any added calories.

This scramble contains only egg whites, but it tastes delicious. If you prefer more protein, just add some cooked chicken breast.

Ingredients:

1 large egg white

1 slice of bread (or toast)

A few leaves of lettuce

Salt and pepper

Preparation: Beat the egg white until stiff peaks form. Toast the bread and spread it with mustard. Top it with the lettuce and scrambled egg white. Season with salt and pepper.

Nutrition Information Calories: 110 kcal Carbohydrates: 10 g Protein: 6 g Fat: 3 g Saturated Fat: 0 g Cholesterol: 15 mg Sodium: 160 mg Potassium: 150 mg Fiber: 1 g Sugar: 1 g Vitamin A: 120 IU Calcium: 45 mg Iron: 1 mg Tried this Recipe? Tag me Today! Mention @ThatGirlCooks-Healthy or tag ThatGirlCooksHealth

4. Peanut Butter Sandwich

Peanuts are rich in monounsaturated fatty acids, which help lower bad LDL cholesterol. They also contain vitamin E, which is useful for skin care.

Ingredients:

2 slices of whole wheat bread

2 teaspoons peanut butter

2 teaspoons jam or jelly

Preparation: Spread the peanut butter onto both sides of the bread. Add the jam or jelly and place the sandwich back in the fridge for about 5 minutes. Cut the sandwich into halves and enjoy.

Nutrition Information Calorie: 130 kcal Carbs: 16 g Protein: 4 g Fat: 7 g Saturated Fat: 1 g Cholesterol: 0 mg Sodium: 105 mg Potassium: 100 mg Fiber: 2 g Sugar: 2 g Vitamin A: 60 IU Calcium: 25 mg Iron: 1 mg

5. Apple Cinnamon Oatmeal

Apples are very nutritious fruits because they contain many vitamins and minerals such as vitamin C, potassium, manganese, copper, and dietary fiber.

They also contain antioxidants that protect your body from oxidative stress. Oxidative stress occurs when there's too much free radicals in our bodies. Free radicals damage cells, tissues, and organs.

Apples are also known to improve digestion. The pectin found in apples helps break down food in the stomach and release nutrients.

Ingredients:

6 ounces steel-cut oats

1 apple

1 tablespoon cinnamon

1 tablespoon maple syrup

Preparation: Mix all the ingredients together in a bowl. Heat the mixture over medium heat on top of the stove. Cook for about 10 minutes. Serve warm.

Nutrition Information: Calories: 180 Carbs: 27 g Protein: 6 g FAT: 3 g Saturated fat: 1 g Cholesterol 0 mg Sodium: 40 mg Potassium: 320 mg Fiber: 3 g Sugar: 13 g Vitamin A: 80 IU Calcium: 30 mg

6. Yogurt Parfait

Yogurt parfaits are very popular in America. They are made with fresh fruits and yogurt. The combination of yogurt and fruit makes them taste great. These parfaits can be prepared quickly and they are perfect for breakfast.

Ingredients:

- 1 cup plain yogurt

- 2 cups fresh berries (blueberries, strawberries)

- ½ cup granola

Method:

Mix all ingredients together and serve.

Nutrition information: Calories: 250 Carbs: 46 g Protein: 9 g Fat: 8 g Saturated Fat: 2 g Cholesterol: 20 mg Sodium: 90 mg Potassium: 400 mg Fiber: 12 g Sugar: 21 g Vitamin A: 50 IU Calcium: 125 mg Iron: 3 mg Tried this Recipe? Tag me Today!

7. Banana Nut Bread

Bananas are one of the best sources of potassium. It has been shown that eating bananas reduces blood pressure and improves heart health. Bananas also have anti-inflammatory properties.

Ingredients:

3/4 cup flour

½ teaspoon baking soda

¼ teaspoon baking powder

¾ teaspoon ground cinnamon

Pinch of nutmeg

Pinch of salt

1 ripe banana

1 egg

1 tablespoon vegetable oil

1 tablespoon honey

1 tablespoon milk

Preparation: Preheat oven to 350 degrees F. Grease an 8x8 inch pan with nonstick cooking spray. In a large bowl, combine dry ingredients. Mash the banana well. Beat the egg and add it to the mashed banana. Stir in oil, honey, and milk. Pour batter into greased pan. Bake at 350°F for 30–35 minutes until golden brown. Let cool completely before cutting.

Nutrition Information Calories: 150 Carbs: 26 g Protein: 3 g Fat: 5 g Saturated Fat: 0 g Cholesterol: 15 mg Sodium: 110 mg Potassium: 230 mg

8. Egg White Muffins

Egg whites are rich in protein and low in calories. They provide essential amino acids which help build muscles and bones. They are also high in iron.

Ingredients:

2 eggs

1/3 cup sugar

1/3 cup white whole wheat flour

1/3 cup oat bran

1/3 cup flax seed meal

1 teaspoon baking soda

1/2 teaspoon salt

Preparation: Combine all the ingredients in a blender or food processor. Blend until smooth. Spoon the batter into muffin tins lined with paper liners. Bake at 375 degrees F for 18–20 minutes or until lightly browned. Remove from pans immediately after removing from the oven. Cool slightly before serving.

Nutrition Information; Calories: 120 Carbs: 17 g Protein: 7 g Fat: 4 g Saturated Fat: 1 g Cholesterol: 55 mg Sodium: 240 mg Potassium: 170 mg

9. Oatmeal Raisin Cookies

Oatmeal is a good source of fiber and it helps lower cholesterol levels. It contains antioxidants which protect against cancer. This cookie recipe uses oats instead of flour.

Ingredients:

1 cup rolled oats

1/3 cup butter

1/3 cup packed brown sugar

1/3 teaspoon salt

1/3 cup molasses

1 egg

1 teaspoon vanilla extract

1/3 cup raisins

Preparation: Melt butter in a saucepan. Add remaining ingredients except raisins. Mix thoroughly. Drop by spoonfuls onto ungreased cookie sheets. Sprinkle with raisins. Bake at 350 degrees F for 10–12 minutes. Allow cookies to cool on racks.

Nutrition Information: Calories: 140 Carbs: 16 g Protein: 3 g Total Fat: 6 g Saturated Fat: 3 g Cholesterol: 40 mg Sodium: 95 mg Potassium: 60 mg

10. Peanut Butter Brownies

Peanuts contain many nutrients like vitamin E, magnesium, folate, copper, zinc, and manganese. They are also a good source of fiber. Peanuts are also a good source for monounsaturated fats.

Ingredients:

6 tablespoons unsalted peanut butter

2 tablespoons cocoa powder

½ cup granulated sugar

¼ cup light brown sugar

1 egg

2 teaspoons vanilla extract

1½ cups flour

1 teaspoon baking powder

½ teaspoon salt

½ cup chopped peanuts

Preparation: Heat oven to 350 degrees F and grease an 8 x 8-inch square baking dish. In a medium bowl, whisk together the peanut butter, both sugars, egg, and vanilla. Whisk in the flour, baking powder, and salt. Fold in the nuts. Spread the mixture evenly in the prepared baking dish. Bake for 25–30 minutes or until set. Cut into squares while still warm. Serve plain or top with chocolate chips.

Gut Health Lunch Recipes

Gut health lunch recipes

Are you looking for healthy gut health lunch recipes? Then you are at right place. Here I am going to share with you some delicious gut health lunch recipes that will give you energy throughout the day.

These healthy gut health lunch recipes are very easy to make. You can prepare them within 30 minutes. If you want to learn more about how to eat healthy then you should read my article on How To Eat Healthy.

Here are the best gut health lunch recipes for this week. Try these out and let me know what do you think about them.

1. Spicy Indian Lentil Soup

This spicy lentil soup is perfect for those who love spicy foods. The spices used in this soup include ginger garlic paste, cumin, coriander seeds, turmeric, red chili pepper, garam masala, and black pepper. All these spices have anti-inflammatory properties. These spices help reduce inflammation caused due to stress and anxiety.

This soup has a rich taste and it is loaded with protein. So, if you are looking for a quick meal then try this one.

Ingredients:

2 cups lentils (red)

4 cups water

8 cloves of garlic

1 tablespoon ginger

1 small onion

2 green chilies

1 teaspoon cumin seeds

1 teaspoon coriander seeds

1 teaspoon turmeric

1 teaspoon red chili pepper flakes

1 teaspoon garam masala

Black pepper

Salt as per taste

Preparation: Wash the lentils under running tap water. Drain well. Put all the ingredients in a pressure cooker. Cook for 5 whistles. Remove from heat. Let it stand for 15 mins. Blend using hand blender. Garnish with fresh coriander leaves.

Nutrition Information

Calories: 250 Carbs: 45 g Protein: 14 g Total Fat: 4 g Saturated Fat: 1 g Cholesterol: 0 mg Sodium: 130 mg Potassium: 740 mg

2. Vegetable Stir Fry

Vegetables are full of vitamins and minerals. This stir fry recipe is made up of vegetables such as broccoli, cauliflower, carrots, peas, beans, cabbage, spinach, mushrooms, zucchini, and tomatoes. It contains no meat but it tastes great.

Ingredients:

1 large head of broccoli

3 medium sized cauliflowers

5 carrots

1 bunch spring onions

1/2 cup frozen peas

1 cup baby corn

1 cup kidney beans

1 cup shredded cabbage

1 cup sliced mushrooms

1 cup diced zucchini

1 tomato

1/2 tsp crushed red chilli flakes

1/2 tsp ground cumin

1 tbsp olive oil

1/2 tsp sea salt

1/2 tsp freshly cracked black pepper

Preparation: Peel the skin off the carrot and cut into 2 inch pieces. Slice the broccoli florets lengthwise. Slice the cauliflower into bite size pieces. Peel the stem of the broccoli and slice into thin strips. Slice the spring onions into rings. Slice the mushrooms into slices. Dice the zucchini into cubes. Chop the baby corn. Rinse the beans. Boil the kettle. Heat the oil in a wok or frying pan over high heat. Add the chopped spring onions and saute until slightly browned. Add the broccoli and cook for 3 minutes. Add the cauliflower and carrots. Saute for another 3 minutes. Add the peas, beans, cabbage and mushrooms. Mix well. Season with salt and pepper. Continue cooking for an additional minute. Add the tomato and mix well. Sprinkle with crushed red chilli flakes and cumin. Serve hot.

Nutrition Information: Calories: 168 Carbs: 32 g Protein: 8 g Total Fat: 6 g Saturated Fat: 2 g Cholesterol: 0mg Sodium: 300 mg Potassium: 990 mg

3. Chicken Korma

Chicken korma is a delicious Indian dish. It is spiced with coriander powder, cinnamon, cardamom, clove, nutmeg, and mace. The chicken is cooked in yogurt and coconut milk along with other spices.

Ingredients:

6 boneless chicken thighs

1/2 tsp turmeric

1/2 tsp cayenne pepper

1/2 tsp paprika

1/4 tsp cumin powder

1/4 tsp fenugreek seeds

1/4 tsp caraway seeds

1/4 cup plain yogurt

1/4 cup unsweetened desiccated coconut

1/4 cup light cream

1/4 cup water

1/2 tsp salt

1/4 tsp freshly ground black pepper

1/4 tsp ground ginger

1/4 tsp garlic paste

1/2 tsp onion powder

1/2 tsp dried mint

1/2 tsp garam masala

1/8 tsp ground cloves

Preparation: Preheat oven to 400 degrees F (200 degrees C). Grease a baking sheet. Cut each thigh into two pieces. Place on prepared baking sheet. Bake for 10-12 minutes or until golden brown. Set aside. In a small bowl combine the yogurt, coconut, cream, water, salt, and pepper. Whisk well. Combine the remaining ingredients in a food processor. Process until smooth. Pour mixture over the chicken. Bake for 20 minutes. Remove from oven. Let stand 5 minutes before serving.

Nutrition Information Per Serving: Calories: 476 Carbs: 15 g Protein: 41 g Total Fat: 26 g Saturated Fat: 12 g Cholesterol: 103 mg Sodium: 767 mg Potassium: 487 mg

4. Ginger Beef Soup

This soup is made using beef broth, fresh ginger root, lemongrass, and green chilies. This spicy soup is perfect when you are feeling under the weather.

Ingredients:

2 tablespoons vegetable oil

2 cups thinly sliced shallots

2 teaspoons minced garlic

1 teaspoon minced fresh gingerroot

1 tablespoon minced lemongrass

1/2 pound lean beef stew meat

1 quart beef broth

1 can (14 ounces) petite diced tomatoes

1/2 jalapeno chili

1/4 cup heavy whipping cream

1/4 teaspoon sugar

Salt to taste

Freshly ground black pepper to taste

Preparation: Heat oil in large saucepan over medium heat. Add shallots and garlic; saute 1 minute. Stir in ginger, lemongrass and beef; saute about 5 minutes or until beef is no longer pink. Drain any fat. Stir in broth, tomatoes, jalapeno chili, and sugar. Bring to boil. Reduce heat to low; cover and simmer 30 minutes. Puree soup in blender or food processor until very smooth. Return to pot. Stir in cream. Cook over medium heat, stirring occasionally, until heated through. Season with salt and black pepper. Serves 4.

Nutrition Information per serving: Calories: 173 Carbohydrates: 11 g Protein: 18 g Fat: 11 g Saturated Fat: 4 g Cholesterol: 55 mg Sodium: 543 mg Potassium: 635 mg

5. Roasted Red Pepper Soup

Roasting red peppers brings out their natural sweetness. They also become soft and tender. If you want to make this recipe healthier, use canned roasted red peppers instead of raw ones.

Ingredients:

1 tablespoon olive oil

1/2 yellow onion, chopped

1 carrot, peeled and chopped

1 celery stalk, chopped

1 bay leaf

1/2 teaspoon kosher salt

1/4 teaspoon freshly ground black pepper

2 pounds Roma tomatoes, seeded and chopped

2 garlic cloves, minced

2 cups vegetable stock

1 cup dry white wine

1/2 cup roasted red bell peppers, drained and coarsely chopped

1/2 cup heavy cream

1/4 cup grated Parmesan cheese

Preparation: In a Dutch oven, heat oil over medium-high heat. Add onions and carrots; cook, stirring frequently, 3 minutes. Add celery and bay leaf; season with salt and pepper. Cover and reduce heat to medium. Cook, stirring often, 8 minutes. Uncover and add tomatoes, garlic, and stock; bring to a boil. Reduce heat to medium-low; simmer, uncovered, 25 minutes or until vegetables are softened. Transfer half of tomato mixture to a blender; process until smooth. Return pureed mixture to pot along with wine. Increase heat to high; return mixture to a boil. Reduce to a simmer; cover and cook 45 minutes or until flavors blend. Remove from heat; stir in roasted peppers and cream. Serve sprinkled with cheese. Makes 10 servings.

Nutrition information per serving: Calories: 125 Carbohydrates: 9 g Protein: 2 g Fat: 6 g Saturated Fat: 3 g Cholesterol: 16 mg Sodium: 221 mg Potassium: 554 mg

6. Spicy Black Bean Chili

Black beans have been used for centuries as a staple food in many cultures around the world. It has been found that they contain more protein than other types of legumes. The spices in this recipe give it an amazing flavor.

Ingredients:

3 tablespoons olive oil

1 small sweet onion, finely chopped

2 garlic cloves

1/2 teaspoon crushed red pepper flakes

1 (15 ounce) can black beans, rinsed and drained

1 (14.5 ounce) can diced tomatoes

1 (8 ounce) can tomato sauce

1 (4 ounce) can green chiles, drained

1 teaspoon cumin

1/2 teaspoon coriander

salt and freshly ground black pepper

1/4 cup chopped fresh cilantro

Preparation: Preheat oven to 350 degrees F. Place all ingredients except cilantro into a bowl and mix well. Pour into a greased 13x9 inch baking dish. Bake, covered, 35 minutes. Sprinkle with cilantro before serving. Makes 6 servings.

Nutrition Information Per Serving: Calories: 171 Carbohydrates: 22 g Protein: 7 g Fat: 7 g Saturated Fat: 1 g Cholesterol: 0 mg Sodium: 576 mg Potassium: 590 mg

7. Curried Lentil Soup

Curries are one of my favorite dishes to eat. This soup is delicious because of its unique combination of curry powder, coconut milk, and lentils. You may substitute brown rice for the quinoa if you prefer.

Ingredients:

2 teaspoons olive oil

1 large onion, chopped

1 large carrot, chopped

1 rib celery, chopped

1 clove garlic, minced

1 pound lean ground beef

1/2 teaspoon turmeric

1/2 teaspoon curry powder

1/2 teaspoon chili powder

1/2 teaspoon dried thyme

1 tablespoon tomato paste

1 cup uncooked quinoa

1 (13.5 ounce) can light coconut milk

1 (16 ounce) can kidney beans, rinsed

1 (14.75 ounce) can fire-roasted diced tomatoes

1 (10 ounce) can condensed tomato soup

1/2 cup water

1/2 cup frozen peas

salt and freshly cracked black pepper

Preparation: Heat oil in a large skillet over medium heat. Add onion, carrot, and celery; saute 4 minutes or until tender. Stir in garlic and next seven ingredients (through tomato paste). Bring to a boil; reduce heat to low. Simmer 15 minutes or until meat is no longer pink. Meanwhile, place quinoa in a fine mesh strainer set over a bowl. Rinse under cold running water; drain well. Stir quinoa into meat mixture; transfer to a slow cooker. Combine remaining ingredients in a microwaveable container. Microwave on High 30 seconds or until hot. Pour over meat mixture, stirring gently to combine. Cover and cook on Low 6 hours. Makes 6 servings. Nutrition information per serving: Calories 248 Carbohydrates 29 g Protein 23 g Fat 11 g Saturated Fat 5 g Cholesterol 57 mg Sodium 624 mg Potassium 828 mg

8. Beef and Broccoli Stir Fry

This healthy version of Chinese takeout includes broccoli instead of white rice. A great way to get kids to eat their vegetables!

Ingredients:

1 pound flank steak

2 tablespoons soy sauce

2 tablespoons sesame oil

2 tablespoons honey

1 tablespoon cornstarch

1 tablespoon vegetable oil

1 head broccoli, cut into florets

1/2 red bell pepper, thinly sliced

1/4 cup chicken broth

In a shallow bowl, whisk together soy sauce, sesame oil, honey, and cornstarch. Cut flank steak across grain into thin strips. In a wok or large nonstick skillet, heat vegetable oil over high heat. Add beef; stir fry 3 minutes or until cooked through. Remove from pan. Drain any excess fat. Add broccoli to pan; stir-fry 2 minutes. Transfer broccoli to a plate. Add bell pepper to pan; stir-fried 3 minutes or until crisp-tender. Return beef to pan; add soy sauce mixture and broth. Cook and stir until thickened. Serve with broccoli. Makes 4 servings.

Nutrition information per serving: Calories: 245 Carbohydrates: 12 g Protein: 18 g Fat: 10 g Saturated Fat: 3 g Cholesterol: 76 mg Sodium: 912 mg Potassium: 201 mg

9. Chicken and Corn Soup

A super simple recipe that's perfect for lunch or dinner. The best part about this recipe is that it takes less than five minutes to make!

Ingredients:

3 cups chicken stock

2 boneless skinless chicken breasts

1 small yellow squash, cubed

1 zucchini, cubed

1/2 sweet potato, peeled and cubed

1/4 cup fresh cilantro leaves

1 lime, juiced

Salt and freshly ground black pepper

Heat oven to 400 degrees F. Place chicken breasts between two pieces of plastic wrap. Using a mallet or rolling pin, flatten chicken breasts to 1/4 inch thickness. Season both sides of each breast with salt and pepper. Place chicken on a baking sheet lined with parchment paper. Bake 20 minutes or until done. Let cool slightly, then shred chicken using two forks. Set aside. To the same pan used to bake chicken, add squash, zucchini, and sweet potatoes. Sprinkle with salt and pepper. Roast until tender, about 25 minutes. Meanwhile, bring chicken stock to a simmer in a medium saucepan. Reduce heat to low. When squash is tender, remove from oven. Add squash to stock along with cilantro and lime juice. Whisk soup until smooth. Divide among bowls and top with shredded chicken. Serves 4. Nutrition Information: Serving Size: 1 cup | Calories: 158 | Fat: 7 grams | Carbs: 13 grams

Fiber: 2 grams

Protein: 19 grams

Sodium: 533 milligrams

10. Turkey Meatball Sub

The secret ingredient here is kalamata olives. They give these sub sandwiches an extra kick of flavor without adding too much sodium.

Ingredients:

6 ounces lean turkey sausage, casing removed

1 egg, lightly beaten

1 teaspoon dried oregano

1/2 cup panko breadcrumbs

1/2 cup grated Parmesan cheese

1/2 teaspoon kosher salt

1/4 teaspoon freshly ground black pepper

1/2 cup olive oil

1/2 cup Italian dressing

4 whole wheat hoagie buns, split

1/2 pound thinly sliced deli ham

4 slices provolone cheese

1/2 cup baby arugula

Preheat oven to 350°F. Line a baking sheet with parchment paper. Heat a cast-iron skillet over medium-high heat. Working in batches, cook sausages 6 to 8 minutes or until browned, turning occasionally. Transfer to prepared baking sheet. Bake 15 minutes or until heated through. While sausages are cooking, combine egg, oregano, breadcrumbs, Parmesan, salt, and pepper in a shallow dish. Mix well. Heat oil in a large skillet over medium-high. Dip meatballs in egg mixture, allowing excess to drip off. Roll in crumb mixture. Return to skillet; cook 5 minutes or until golden. Remove from skillet. Spread half of dressing onto bottom halves of hoagie buns. Top with sausages, ham, and cheese. Spoon remaining dressing over sandwiches. Arrange arugula evenly on top. Cover with bun tops. Makes 4 servings. Nutrition Information: Serving size: 1 sandwich

Calories: 397

Fat: 30 grams

Carbs: 26 grams

Fiber: 1 gram

Protein: 28 grams

Sodium: 912 milligrams

Gut Health Dinner Recipes

Are you looking for healthy dinner recipes? This section has all kinds of delicious and nutritious recipes. We also provide information regarding health and nutrition.

Healthy food is very important for our guts to stay fit and active. In order to keep ourselves fit and healthy we need to eat right food. Eating healthy food is not only good for our body but also for our mind. When we eat right food we feel happy and energetic.

We have shared some of the most delicious and nutritious recipes with you. These recipes are easy to cook and taste great. This section has been designed keeping in mind the needs of everyone.

So, let's check out the following recipes and enjoy eating healthy food.

1) Chicken Soup with Kale and Cabbage

Ingredients:

• 1 chicken breast (cut into pieces)

• 2 cups of water

• ½ cup of kale leaves (chopped)

• ¼ cup of cabbage (finely chopped)

• Salt as per taste

Method:

Cook the chicken in boiling water until tender. Add salt and let it cool down. Remove the bones and shred the meat. In a large pot add the shredded chicken along with the vegetables. Cook till they turn soft. Serve hot.

2) Spicy Indian Salad

This is one of my favorite salad recipes because it's very easy to make and tastes great! It can be served as a main meal or snack. This recipe contains all the essential nutrients which are required by the body. The combination of different spices gives this salad a spicy flavor.

Ingredients:

• 3 cups of mixed greens (washed and dried)

- 1/3 cup of red onion (thinly sliced)

- 1 tomato (diced)

- 1 cucumber (peeled, seeded, and diced)

- ½ cup of fresh coriander leaves (finely chopped) – optional

- 1 green chili (seeded and finely chopped) – optional

- 1 tablespoon of cumin powder

- 1 tablespoon of turmeric powder

- 1 tablespoon fenugreek seeds

- 1 tablespoon of paprika

- 1 tablespoon of garam masala

- 1 tablespoon of ginger paste

- 1 tablespoon of garlic paste

- 1 tablespoon lime juice

- 1 tablespoon of lemon juice

- 1 teaspoon of salt

- 1 teaspoon of sugar

- 2 tablespoons of olive oil

- 1/4 cup of plain yogurt

Method:

Mix all the ingredients together except the yogurt. Let it rest at room temperature for about an hour so that the flavors get blended properly. Once done stir in the yogurt. If you want more spice then add more ginger and garlic paste. You may use less if you do not like too much spiciness.

3) Mediterranean Quinoa Salad

This is another simple but tasty salad that I love making during summer time. It has lots of veggies, grains, herbs, and nuts. All these ingredients give it a complete protein rich nutrition.

Ingredients:

– 1 cup of quinoa

– 1 carrot (cubed)

– 1 zucchini (slice lengthwise)

– 1 small yellow bell pepper (thinly slice)

– 1 cup of cherry tomatoes (halved)

– 1/2 cup of feta cheese (shredded)

– 1/4 cup of mint leaves (chopped) – optional

– 2 tablespoons of basil leaves (chopped) -optional

– 1 tablespoon of oregano leaves (chopped)– optional

– 1 clove of garlic (minced)

– 1 tablespoon of white vinegar

– 1/2 teaspoon of salt

– Black pepper as per taste

– Olive oil as needed

Method:

In a medium sized bowl combine all the ingredients except the black pepper, olive oil, and vinegar. Mix well. Cover and place in the fridge overnight. When ready serve chilled. Garnish with extra herbs if desired.

4) Lentil Rice Pilaf

I have included lentils in this rice pilaf recipe because they are high in fiber and low in fat. They help in digestion and reduce cholesterol levels. This dish is perfect for lunch box or dinner party.

Ingredients:

1) 1 cup of basmati rice

2) 1 cup of brown lentils (soaked in plenty of water for 6 hours)

3) 1 cup of carrots (cut into cubes)

4) 1 cup of cauliflower florets (cut into cubes) – optional

5) 1 cup of peas (shelled) – optional

6) 1/2 teaspoon of turmeric powder

7) 1/2 teaspoon cayenne pepper

8) 1/2 teaspoon cinnamon powder

9) 1 teaspoon of ground cumin

10) Salt as per taste

11) 2 tablespoons of olive oil – optional

12) Lemon juice as per taste

13) Water as needed

14) Garlic cloves (crushed)

15) Chopped parsley as garnish

Method:

Cook the rice according to instructions on the package. In a large pan heat the olive oil and saute the onions until golden brown. Add the crushed garlic and cook for few seconds. Stir in the spices and fry for few minutes. Now add the vegetables and saute till soft. Finally pour in the cooked rice and mix well. Season with salt and pepper. Serve hot sprinkled with chopped parsley.

5) Chickpeas & Spinach Curry

Chickpeas are one of my favorite legumes. They are loaded with nutrients like iron, zinc, folate, magnesium, calcium, B vitamins, etc. So when I came across this curry recipe I had to try it out immediately. The chickpeas provide a good source of protein while spinach adds some green color to the curry.

Ingredients:

• 1 can of chickpeas (drained and rinsed)

- 1 onion – cut into wedges

- 4 cloves of garlic – minced

- 2-3 fresh red chilies – finely sliced

- 1 teaspoon of grated ginger

- 1/2 teaspoon of garam masala powder

- 1/2 cup of tomato puree

- 1/2 tsp. turmeric powder

- 1/4 tsp. chili powder

- 1 teaspoon of coriander powder

- 3 cups of baby spinach

- 1 tbsp. lemon juice

- Salt as per taste

- Oil as required

- Fresh cilantro as garnish

Method :

Heat up half a cup of oil in a deep skillet over medium heat. Add the onions and saute till golden. Add the garlic, ginger, and spices and stir for a minute. Then add the tomato puree and let it simmer for 5 minutes. Turn off the heat and keep aside. Heat the remaining oil in another skillet and saute the spinach until wilted. Remove from heat and set aside. In a food processor blend the chickpeas along with the spinach, tomatoes, and lemon juice. Pour the contents back into the same skillet. Let it come to room temperature. If you want more flavor then sprinkle some freshly roasted cashews on top. Sprinkle with cilantro leaves and serve warm.

6) Vegetable Stir-Fry

One of the easiest ways to eat healthy is by making vegetable dishes at home. When I was growing up my mom used to make stir fries all the time. She would chop veggies really fine and use them to make delicious meals. Here's a simple version of her style of cooking. You can use any kind of vegetables that you have available.

Ingredients:

- 1 bunch of broccoli – cut into small pieces

- 1 medium sized carrot – peeled and cut into thin strips

- 1 zucchini – cut into thick slices

- 1 yellow squash – cut into thin slices

- 1 bell pepper – cut into long strips

- 1 tablespoon of olive oil

- 1 clove of garlic – minced

- 1/2 tsp. black pepper

- 1/2 tsp. salt

- 1/8 tsp. nutmeg

- 1/8 cup of water or stock

– 1/2 cup of frozen peas

– 1/2 green cabbage – shredded

– 1/2 bunch of kale – shredded

Preparation:

Heat up the olive oil in a wok or big saucepan. Saute the garlic for about 30 seconds. Add the rest of the ingredients except the cabbage and kale. Cook everything together for about 10 minutes. Then add the cabbage and kale. Cover and cook for 5 minutes. Uncover and toss gently. Serve hot.

7) Coconut Rice

This is an easy way to eat coconut without having to go through the hassle of frying it. It tastes great too!

Ingredients:

• 2 cups of basmati rice

• 1/2 large sweet potato – peeled and cubed

• 1 inch piece of ginger – thinly sliced

• 1/2 lime – juiced

• 1/2 ripe mango – chopped

• 1 can of full fat coconut milk

• 1/2 tbsp. sugar

• 1/2 jalapeno – seeded and diced

• 1/2 red capsicum – deseeded and chopped

- 1/2 green capsicum – deseed and chopped

- Salt as per preference

- Fresh cilantro leaves – chopped

Preparation: Boil the rice for 20 minutes. Drain excess water. Mix all the other ingredients in a bowl. Put the cooked rice in this mixture and mix well. Garnish with fresh cilantro leaves.

8) Lentils with Carrots

Lentils are one of the best sources of protein when compared to meat. They contain lots of fiber which helps control blood sugar levels. This dish is perfect if you are looking to lose weight or just need something filling after a workout.

Ingredients:

- 1 cup of lentils – soaked overnight

- 1 cup of carrots – grated

- 1 onion – finely chopped

- 1 inch piece ginger – grated

- 4 cloves of garlic – minced

- 1/2 cup of curry powder

- 1/2 teaspoon cinnamon

- 1/4 teaspoon ground turmeric

- 1/4 cup of water

- 3 tablespoons of sunflower oil

- Salt as per taste

- 1/4 tsp. garam masala

- 1/4 red chili – chopped

- 1/4 green chili – chopped

- Fresh coriander leaves – chopped

Prepared: Soak the lentils for 8 hours. Rinse thoroughly and drain. Keep the soaking liquid. Grate the carrots and slice the onion. Peel and mince the garlic. Chop the ginger. Combine the lentils, carrots, onion, garlic, ginger, and spice powders in a pan. Add the water and bring to boil. Reduce heat and cover. Simmer for 15-20 minutes until soft. Heat the oil in another pan. Fry the spices for about 2 minutes. Add the onions and fry for about 6 more minutes. Add the garlic and fry for another minute. Add the tomatoes and simmer for about 10 minutes. Now add the carrots and lentils. Bring back to boil and then simmer covered for about 10 minutes until the lentils are tender. Season with salt and serve garnished with fresh coriander leaves.

9) Quinoa Salad

Quinoa has been gaining popularity among people who want to follow a gluten free diet. The reason why quinoa is so popular is because it contains high amounts of protein and low calories. If you are on a ketogenic diet, quinoa is also considered a good source of fats. In fact, it is even higher than flax seeds.

Ingredients:

1 cup of quinoa

3 cups of vegetable broth

1/4 cup of lemon juice

2 medium sized tomatoes – chopped

1 small cucumber – chopped

1/2 bunch of parsley – chopped

1/4 cup extra virgin olive oil

Salt and pepper to taste

Prepared: Wash the quinoa thoroughly. Boil the quinoa and let it cool down completely. Once cooled, transfer into a salad bowl. Pour the stock over the quinoa and set aside. In a blender, blend the remaining ingredients until smooth. Pour this dressing over the quinoa. Toss well and enjoy immediately.

10) Baked Eggplant Dinner

Eggplants have always been associated with being healthy. However, many people avoid eating eggplants due to their bitter taste. But, there's no need to worry anymore! You can easily prepare delicious dishes using eggplants without having to worry about its bitterness. This baked eggplant dinner is perfect for those who don't like spicy food but still love Indian flavors.

Ingredients:

– 1 large eggplant – cut lengthwise

– 1 tablespoon of tandoori paste

– Salt as per taste

– Lemon juice

– Garlic – crushed

– Onion – sliced

– Red chilli – chopped

Prepared : Cut the eggplant into half lengthwise. Place the pieces in an oven tray lined with aluminum foil. Sprinkle some salt on top of the eggplant and bake at 350 degrees F for 30 minutes or until cooked through. Remove from the oven and drizzle with lemon juice. Mix together all the other ingredients and spread evenly over the eggplant halves. Bake again for another 5 minutes. Serve hot.

11) Avocado Soup

Avocados are one of the best sources of monounsaturated fatty acids (MUFAs). These oils help reduce cholesterol levels and prevent heart diseases. They are also rich in vitamin E, potassium, magnesium, folate, thiamine, riboflavin, niacin, pantothenic acid, copper, phosphorus, iron, calcium, fiber, and zinc. It is recommended to consume avocados every day to reap maximum benefits.

Ingredients:

½ avocado – peeled and cubed

¼ teaspoon turmeric powder

¼ teaspoon cumin powder

One litre of chicken stock

A few sprigs of mint

Pepper

Garnish with freshly grated coconut

Prepared: Blend all the ingredients except the garnish in a blender until smooth. Garnish with freshly grated coconuts before serving.

CHAPTER 13
GUT HEALTH HACKS FOR WOMEN: THE ULTIMATE GUIDE TO A HEALTHY GUT

WOMEN TEND to be more sensitive than men to changes in their gut. When women go through hormonal shifts — before and during menstruation, pregnancy, and menopause — the bacteria (good and bad) in their guts tends to fluctuate more than it does for men. That's why women are generally more likely to experience digestive problems like IBS, bloating, and gas around these times of the year. Furthermore, women also tend to have more trouble with their gut health after giving birth. This is because giving birth can damage your rectal mucous membrane and lower levels of good bacteria. Luckily, there are plenty of things you can do now — and continually throughout your life — to keep a healthy gut that helps you feel amazing every day.

Get to know your gut

Your gut is the part of the digestive system that starts in your mouth and ends at your anus. It is where food is broken down and nutrients are absorbed into your blood. The gut is home to trillions of bacteria that help with digestion, our immune system, and even our moods. There are as many bacterial cells in our gut as there are human cells in our entire body! The health of your gut is key to your overall health. When we're talking gut health, we're really talking about the health of your intestinal tract, which is home to 70% of your immune system. Your gut is where you can change the world. If you are feeding good bacteria, then you are helping to change the world for the better.

Diversify your diet

Diet is one of the most important aspects of gut health. The foods you eat can either help or hinder your digestive system. Eating a variety of foods, including plant-based proteins, natural fats (like avocado, coconut, and olive oil), complex carbs (like sweet potatoes, yams, and brown rice), and plenty of fibrous veggies (like broccoli, asparagus, and green leafy veggies) is one of the best ways to improve your gut health. Another way to improve your gut health is by reducing your intake of processed foods. These often contain high amounts of sugar and other ingredients that can irritate the digestive system. Also, limit or avoid alcohol and caffeine. These can dehydrate your system and worsen digestive issues.

Stress management

Stress can have both short- and long-term effects on your health, including your gut health. It has been shown to increase the production of hormones and neurotransmitters that can cause digestive problems like gas, cramping, and diarrhea. When you're stressed, your body has two options: fight or flight. In times of duress, your body diverts blood flow from less essential organs, like your digestive system, to the muscles to get you out of a dangerous situation. Even if it's just an argument with your significant other, your body reacts the same way and diverts blood from your GI tract to your muscles. Short-term stress — such as getting stuck in traffic — is normal and manageable. However, long-term stress — like dealing with a demanding job or financial burdens — can cause unhealthy and even dangerous changes in your body.

Keep Your Bacteria Happy and Healthy

The best way to do this is by eating a healthy diet. You can also take a probiotic supplement. Studies have shown that probiotics have the power to improve gut health and have many other benefits. Probiotics can help improve digestive symptoms and promote healthy gut bacteria. Another way you can improve the health of your gut bacteria is by eating prebiotic foods. These are high-fiber foods that feed the good bacteria in your gut and are important for a healthy gut. Here are some foods that contain prebiotics: Asparagus Bananas Broccoli Brown rice Chia seeds Flaxseeds Garlic Jerusalem artichoke Leeks Parsnips Radishes Rhubarb

Try a Low-FODMAP Diet

If you've tried everything and your gut health is still suffering, a low-FODMAP diet might be for you. This diet is specifically designed to help people with irritable bowel syndrome (IBS) and other digestive disorders. It's a plan designed to reduce the amount of foods that can cause digestive issues. There are different variations of the low-FODMAP diet, but they all eliminate FODMAPs, which are foods that are high in carbohydrates and can cause digestive issues. FODMAP stands for fermentable oligo-, di-, and monosaccharides and polyols. For example, dairy, legumes, and gluten-free whole grains are high in FODMAPs.

Rotating Proteins, Vegetables, and fiber

We've all heard the saying "eat a balanced diet." But what does that really mean? Well, it means eating a variety of proteins, vegetables, and fiber. Eating a variety of these three aspects of your diet is the best way to keep your gut happy. Different proteins provide different amino acids, which help with the building of muscle and tissue and can also help with mood disorders. Eating a variety of proteins can help prevent deficiency and promote better gut health. Eating a variety of vegetables will also help with gut health since vegetables are high in fiber and nutrients. Fiber is great for your digestive tract and can also help with weight management. Eating a variety of fiber-rich foods is the best way to stay healthy.

Take a Probiotic Supplement

Some people may be lacking in healthy gut bacteria, which can cause digestive problems and lead to other more serious health problems. This can happen after an illness, after taking antibiotics, after a long course of antibiotics, or when your diet is poor. The best way to get these good bacteria back in your gut is to take a probiotic supplement. Probiotics are live microorganisms that are good for your health. They're found in certain types of foods, like yogurt and kefir, and can also be found in supplements. They're often used to treat digestive issues like diarrhea, constipation, and gas. Probiotics also help with other issues like allergies, eczema, and skin problems. They can also help prevent urinary tract infections and vaginal infections. They've also been studied as a treatment for mental health disorders like anxiety and depression.

Light Exercise is Good For Gut Health

Exercising is one of the best things you can do to promote and keep a healthy gut. It can help prevent digestive disorders and promote better immunity. Exercising can also help with weight management, which can improve your digestive system. Exercising can help regulate your digestive system and keep it running smoothly. It can also help with mental health issues such as anxiety and depression, which can also affect your gut health. Exercising regularly can also help with constipation and diarrhea. Note: If you're experiencing diarrhea, avoid exercising until it goes away.

Don't Forget to Breathe!

Taking deep breaths is a great way to help relieve stress and calm your mind and digestive system. This can help prevent digestive issues like diarrhea and constipation. It can also help with feelings of anxiety and depression. When you take a deep breath, you're sending oxygen to your entire body, including your digestive tract. Deep breathing can also be a great way to prevent overeating. Sometimes, when you're stressed or anxious, you may find yourself overeating. Deep breathing before eating can be a great way to prevent this.

Be mindful of what you put in your mouth

As we've discussed, diet is a huge part of gut health. But it doesn't just end with eating the right foods. It's also about eating the right amounts, avoiding trigger foods, and eating at the right times. How much should you eat? Eating the right amount can help balance your blood sugar and prevent digestive issues. Eating too little can actually hurt your immune system and digestive system. Eating too much can cause weight gain, which can also lead to digestive issues. What should you avoid eating?

Foods that are high in fiber can cause digestive issues for some people,

Use Food as Medicine

The best way to use food as medicine is to focus on foods that are high in nutrients and low in sugar. Some examples include:

Foods that are high in antioxidants can help fight inflammation.

Foods that are high in fiber can help you feel full and prevent constipation.

Foods that contain a lot of water help keep your digestive tract running smoothly.

Foods that contain probiotics can help improve your immune system, which will also improve your digestion.

Minimize Stress

Stress is a huge factor when it comes to digestive issues, regardless if you have SIBO or not. Stress has been linked to heart disease, anxiety disorders, depression, weight gain, insomnia and digestive issues. When you're stressed out, your body releases hormones such as cortisol and adrenaline into your blood stream. These hormones can cause inflammation in the digestive tract, which leads to things like bloating and gas. A recent study published in the journal Alimentary Pharmacology & Therapeutics found that psychological stress is associated with gastrointestinal symptoms. In this study, researchers looked at the effects of stress on the gastrointestinal system in 41 healthy volunteers who were exposed to an acute psychological

It's important to find ways to manage your stress so you can avoid unnecessary inflammation in your digestive tract. Try taking up a relaxing hobby like knitting, gardening or walking your dog. You should also consider getting a massage or getting acupuncture treatments on a regular basis. Meditation is also a great way to relax and reduce stress levels. Make time for yourself each day where you can just sit back and do nothing but relax and meditate for 20 minutes or more.

If you have SIBO, then it's especially important to manage your stress because it could make your condition worse if left unmanaged

Why a healthy gut is crucial for women

A healthy gut is crucial for women's health. It's important to maintain a healthy gut flora balance (aka gut microbiome) in order to have a healthy digestive system, to maintain proper immune function, and to help fight off infections and diseases. It's also important for women to have a healthy gut because it can improve their mood and reduce stress levels, which could reduce the chances of developing anxiety and depression. Having an unhealthy gut flora can also contribute to skin problems like acne or eczema, which is another reason why having a healthy gut is crucial for women's health.

There are many factors that can disrupt the balance of bacteria in your gut. Antibiotics, probiotics, processed foods, stress and other negative lifestyle habits can all cause an imbalance in your digestive system that can lead to different health problems down the road. One of the most common causes of an unhealthy gut is consuming too many refined carbohydrates like sugar and flour. Refined carbs can cause a spike in blood sugar, which will then cause your blood sugar to drop, which can make you feel tired and hungry again shortly after eating.

The good news is that there are many ways that women can help improve the health of their gut. By following the ideas in this book, you can help promote the growth of healthy bacteria in your gut.

ABOUT THE AUTHOR

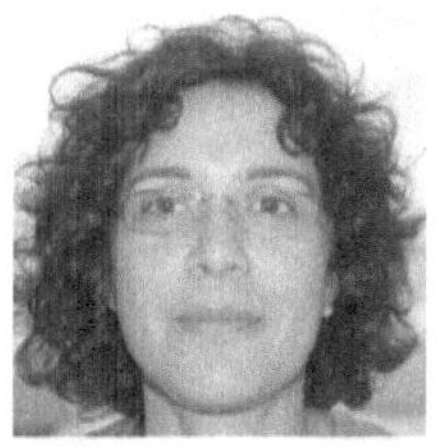

Vanessa Alvarez is an internationally recognized health scientist and author with over 30 years of experience in the field of women's health and wellness, focusing on female digestive health. She studied the female digestive system and microbiome for more than 2 decades, dedicating her life to helping women flourish with natural solutions that are safe for their bodies and minds.

She was born in Seattle, Washington, but raised in Northern California where she spent most of her childhood exploring the outdoors with her family. Nowadays, when not writing or speaking about her work, you can find her enjoying time by herself with her two cats (Chewy and Bacca) or cooking up a storm at home.

www.ingramcontent.com/pod-product-compliance
Lightning Source LLC
Chambersburg PA
CBHW051101250726
48656CB00001B/405